CREATIVE
PHYSICAL ACTIVITIES
AND
EQUIPMENT

CREATIVE
PHYSICAL ACTIVITIES
AND
EQUIPMENT

Bev Davison

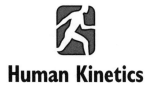

Human Kinetics

Library of Congress Cataloging-In-Publication Data

Davison, Bev. 1957–
    Creative physical activities and equipment / by Bev Davison.
        p. cm.
    Includes bibliographical references (p.) and index.
    ISBN 0-88011-779-6 (paperback)
    1. Sporting goods. 2. Physical education and training--Equipment and supplies.
3. Free material.
    GV745.D38   1998
    796'.028--dc21
                                                            98-11615
                                                            CIP

ISBN: 0-88011-779-6

Copyright © 1998 by Bev Davison

Acquisitions Editor: Scott Wikgren; **Developmental Editor:** Syd Slobodnik; **Assistant Editor:** Katy Patterson; **Copyeditor:** Heather Stith; **Proofreader:** Ann Byler; **Graphic Designer:** Nancy Rasmus; **Graphic Artist:** Joe Bellis; **Cover Designer:** Jack Davis; **Photographer (cover):** Tom Roberts; **Illustrators:** Mary Yemma Long; **Printer:** United Graphics

Human Kinetics books are available at special discounts for bulk purchases. Special editions or book excerpts can also be created to specification. For details, contact the Special Sales Manager at Human Kinetics.

Printed in the United States of America   10   9   8   7   6   5   4   3   2   1

Human Kinetics
Web site: http://www.humankinetics.com/

United States: Human Kinetics, P.O. Box 5076, Champaign, IL 61825-5076
1-800-747-4457
e-mail: humank@hkusa.com

Canada: Human Kinetics, Box 24040, Windsor, ON N8Y 4Y9
1-800-465-7301 (in Canada only)
e-mail: humank@hkcanada.com

Europe: Human Kinetics, P.O. Box IW14, Leeds LS16 6TR, United Kingdom
(44) 1132 781708
e-mail: humank@hkeurope.com

Australia: Human Kinetics, 57A Price Avenue, Lower Mitcham, South Australia 5062
(088) 277 1555
e-mail: humank@hkaustralia.com

New Zealand: Human Kinetics, P.O. Box 105-231, Auckland 1
(09) 523 3462
e-mail: humank@hknewz.com

To my father

Although he did not live to see this published, he would have
been proud.

CONTENTS

CHAPTER 3 SAME OLD STUFF

CHAPTER 4 DON'T THROW IT OUT JUST BECAUSE IT'S BROKEN!

CHAPTER 5 ACQUIRING FREE EQUIPMENT

CHAPTER 6   FUNDRAISING

PREFACE

If you've ever had to stretch a physical education budget to its maximum capacity, this book is for you! Physical education teachers, athletic directors, and recreation directors all know the importance of selecting the most cost-effective equipment that provides the greatest variety while meeting the requirements of educational standards or competitive programs. This book explains how you can make the most out of whatever budget you have for physical education and meet your equipment goals. This book is a vital resource for any physical education program.

This book presents equipment that you can make for a minimum cost. You don't need an elaborate workshop to assemble this equipment; it can be created quickly and easily. This book also provides exciting and fresh games and activities that utilize these pieces of equipment so that you will know how to attain ideal results. The book then explores ways to turn "trash" into great equipment and outlines games and activities employing your new treasures. You will also learn some nontraditional methods of using traditional equipment, which can provide variety in a program without adding costs.

One of the most exciting sections of this book explores how you can acquire free equipment available to schools and nonprofit organizations. Some of these items are available merely by asking for them; other equipment can be traded for proofs of purchases of a product. Generally, no handling fees or postage is required. A section of this book is dedicated to helping you find and acquire the free equipment that is offered.

Finally, creative, yet easy, techniques of raising funds will be presented and described. These fundraising activities are ideal for busy teachers or program administrators because they are not very time-consuming and are easily conducted. Everyone reading this section will find a method of raising money that will be suitable for them and that will fit into their already overcrowded schedules.

This book is organized into three components. The first deals with the making or adapting of equipment. Each creation or adaptation is followed by a game or activity for that piece of equipment. If a program already owns the equipment, the new activity offered for that item may be a refreshing change for the teacher and the students. For example, instructors who have always wanted to teach an activity such as juggling, but have been unable due to the cost factor of the juggling scarves, will be delighted to try adapting old dryer sheets into juggling scarves. Teachers and directors will discover ideas for teaching a variety of activities that have been impossible in the past due to budgetary restraints. Students respond enthusiastically to the new ideas and learning possibilities that will be explored and described in this book.

The second section will be a delightful surprise to many educators who never realized the resources available for free equipment. Methods of obtaining this equipment vary greatly, but with the aid of this book, all teachers and program administrators will be able to enhance program resources for free.

The third section of the book will improve attitudes toward raising funds. These tremendous ideas require a little bit of organizational time, but the dividends compared to the time expended are incredible. Students do not have to sell anything, and fund collection is an easy, uncomplicated process. Soliciting the community for cash is not an element of these fundraising ideas either. These refreshing ideas will be fun for the organizer and for the participants. The parents will be pleased that they will not be asked to financially support another project where they have to consume huge amounts of sugar or other products at a greatly inflated price. Parental support for these projects will be marvelous.

ACKNOWLEDGMENTS

Special thanks to Cathy Porter, whose patience and help have made this book possible. Also thanks to my family who has supported me though this whole endeavor, encouraging me every step of the way.

CHAPTER 1

MAKING EQUIPMENT

Because many physical educators are involved with coaching or other responsibilities, they don't have a lot of time to construct equipment for their programs. The equipment described in this chapter does not require any elaborate plans for construction, nor does it even require a workshop. It has been designed so that even people who are not mechanically inclined can construct it quickly and easily. Also, the materials needed to construct the equipment are very cost-efficient (cheap).

Although most physical educators avoid the industrial arts area of the school (and any other place that can be physically hazardous), you should take a break from the gym and get to know the industrial arts teacher. This person's expertise (and workshop) can be invaluable when you want to construct items of more complexity, such as a miniature golf course for inside the gym. At this level of complexity, the ideas are limitless!

BEAN BAG TARGETS

The possibilities for targets to throw bean bags at range from extremely simple to somewhat complicated. A very simple target to use is old campaign posters. In addition to being readily available and free, campaign posters are usually very durable. They are designed to outlast inclement weather, rocks, and an occasional egg or two, so a few bean bags certainly won't hurt. Simply tape the posters to the walls to use them as targets. Some fun targets can be the current superintendent of schools, school board members, or the mayor. During years when no major election is held, you can duplicate an 8 x 10 picture of an administrator or teacher and post it for targets.

Before you let the children take aim at a poster or picture, however, make sure the people who are pictured agree to having their images used this way. After an election, most candidates will be glad to let anyone take down as many posters as needed to have for targets. (Most will be happy that their name is in front of future voters.) Also, be sure that all political parties are represented so that the activity does not come across as being politically motivated. Finally, before the children take their first toss, explain to them that the target games are all in fun and that no disrespect is intended toward the adults.

You can use milk crates and cans to make another type of target. For example, put steel cans on top of milk crates. To practice underhand throwing, students attempt to throw the bean bags into the crates or the cans. To practice overhand throwing, students attempt to knock over the cans. If you have a lot of cans, make a pyramid of cans. Place the cans in a triangle formation, or stack cans of varying sizes on top of each other. To add some variety, paint the cans a few different colors and assign a different point value to each color. The students can then score points by knocking over the different colored cans. Another extremely easy target that is a favorite of students is a small stuffed animal on top of a milk crate. The younger the students are, the larger the animal should be.

Boxes with holes cut in them also make good targets. You may find old boxes that already have holes in them; for instance, boxes in which balls are packaged often have openings that are just the right size for throwing bean bags into. If you can't find a box with holes, cut holes big enough for bean bags into any large box. Students will enjoy this activity more if you paint a picture, such as a face, on the box and then cut out parts of the picture, such as the eyes, nose, and mouth, to throw the bean bags into.

You can construct a more complicated target from plywood. It would be similar to the cut box, but much more durable. One idea is to paint a clown face on the plywood with the eyes, ears, nose, and mouth cut out. Another possibility is to paint an apple tree on the plywood with some of the apples cut out. You could assign various points to the missing apples to entertain older children.

Finally, you can paint a tic-tac-toe board on a square piece of plywood or cardboard and place it flat on the ground. You can make the board more elaborate by building partitions to divide the board into nine equal squares. The students can toss the bean bags at the board, attempting to play tic-tac-toe. If a bean bag lands into a square that is already occupied, the original bean bag remains and the second is removed from the game. If no tic-tac-toe formation is made, the student with the most bean bags on the board is the winner of the round.

PLASTIC BOTTLE EQUIPMENT

Old plastic bottles can be a great asset to any physical education program. The best ones are the gallon bottles in which vinegar or sugar-sweetened drinks are packaged. They resemble bleach bottles, but do not contain any residue that may be potentially hazardous to students. You can also use gallon or half-gallon milk containers. You can use these bottles in their original form or cut into a variety of pieces of equipment to be used throughout the year. Keeping several empty bottles stored away for later or for emergency use is a great idea. (Note: These bottles should be thoroughly rinsed with water and left without their caps for two or three days to eliminate any sugar residue before they are resealed for use in the gym.)

AREA MARKERS

You can use bottles that are in good condition for area markers. They serve the same purposes as more expensive traffic cones that are sold through equipment companies. For each area marker, one empty bottle and some water or sand is necessary. The bottles will stay in place if they are filled approximately half full with water. Less sand is required to secure bottles, but sand is usually more difficult to fill the bottles with and is not always as readily available as water. You may want to paint the bottles with spray paint to help you color-code groups for activities. For instance, each group could report to a different area that would be marked by color-specific plastic bottles.

WEIGHTS

You can use plastic bottles that are partially filled with water or sand as weights for aerobics workouts or to carry while walking or jogging. You can also fill plastic bottles to various degrees for use in weight training. Students can lift one bottle at a time, or you can put two bottles on the ends of a PVC pipe or broom handle to make a barbell for lifting. The easiest way to do this is to put the PVC pipe through the handles of the plastic bottles and tie the bottles to the pipe with rope or cord. To make the bottles more secure, drill a hole through the pipe and thread the rope or cord through it. Although younger children should not lift these weights, children in the fourth grade or higher can be introduced to some strength development in this fashion.

SCOOPS

You can cut off the bottoms of the plastic bottles either at an angle or straight across to make scoops to use for digging or catching (figure 1.1). The scoops are great to use to practice catching with the nondominant hand, as is done in softball and baseball. The students can play T-ball using a tennis ball and scoops instead of gloves for the outfielders.

To make a hand-eye coordination activity from the scoops, punch a hole in the cap of the scoop and lace a piece of cord inside. The cord should be approximately 18 to 24 inches in length. Tie a knot in the cord so that it remains secure inside the scoop and replace the cap. Tie the other end of the cord to a small Wiffle ball. The students toss the ball into the air and attempt to catch it with the scoop. With this piece of equipment, students do not have to run all over the gym to recover a ball that is not caught, which gives them more time to spend on the activity and prevents traffic jams in the gym.

SCOOP BALL

Scoop Ball is a fast-moving game that uses the scoops made from plastic bottles and a tennis ball. Because this game moves fast, you should cover the edges of the scoops with a heavy tape, such as duct tape, in order to prevent possible injury to the students. Each player has a scoop, and each team has a goal line at opposite ends of the gym.

The object of the game is to get the ball across the goal line by throwing it to players on your team. You may want to divide the gym into playing areas with area markers so that several groups can play at the same time. The teams should have three or four players per team.

Start the game at the center of the court. To determine which team has first possession of the ball, you can flip a coin, or you can bounce the ball high and let one player from each team scramble for it. The player who recovers the ball gains possession for the team. To move the ball across the gym, players must toss it from their scoops. A player who has the ball in her scoop may not move; all other players may move. The penalty for walking with the ball is three giant steps away from the opponent's goal line. A player on the other team may intercept a pass with his or her scoop. Players may not touch the ball with their hands. To pick up the ball from the floor, a player must use the scoop. If a player touches the ball with his hand, the ball is given to a player on the other team.

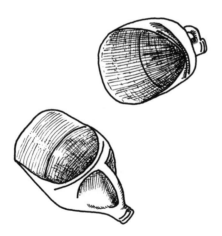

Figure 1.1 Scoops

TAMBOURINES

Save the bottoms of the plastic bottles that you cut to make scoops. You can use these bottoms to make tambourines that the children can play when participating in rhythm activities or dancing. These instruments add an extra dimension of coordination to the dance or rhythmic movement. The students may merely shake them while participating or may move them to the rhythm of the music. The students also may bang them against the hip or the hand at a specific point during a dance.

To make the tambourines, punch holes every two inches around the bottom of the bottle, approximately an inch away from the edge. A heavy-duty hole puncher should be able to do this. Using pipe cleaners, tie together two large metallic washers and tie them to the hole in the bottom of the bottle. Each hole should have two washers attached when the tambourine is completed. Trim any excess pipe cleaner so that no pipe cleaners are loose or poking out from the tambourine. The washers hit each other as the tambourine is moved and make a clinking noise.

STORAGE CONTAINERS

You can make wonderful storage containers by cutting off the top of a plastic bottle. These containers are perfect for storing small items such as bean bags, marbles, or balloons.

STREAMERS

Streamers are an exciting addition to a physical education program whether they are very simply made or made with more time-consuming methods. Possibly the simplest streamers to make are garbage bags that are cut into two-inch strips. You can cut the bags with a paper cutter to form even edges, but scissors will also work. Streamers cut with scissors will be a little more jagged around the edges. Cut the bags along the length for older children or along the width for younger children. Children hold the end of the bag and wave it as a streamer.

You can make a more complicated, yet more colorful, version of the streamers using a 12-inch dowel rod, an eyelet screw, a fishing swivel, and 6 to 10 feet of ribbon that is two inches wide. Screw the eyelet screw into the end of the dowel rod. Attach one end of the fishing swivel to the eyelet. Fold one end of the ribbon over approximately half an inch and sew it down. Then lace the other end of the fishing swivel through the hole that is created by sewing the edge of the ribbon down. The other end of the ribbon should also be sewn down or cut with pinking shears to keep the ribbon from fraying.

You can use the streamers with music to develop creative movement or to form a routine that a group can perform. Be sure each student has plenty of space, in order to prevent children from being hit by other streamers. Some streamer actions include the following:

- *Large circles.* Move the streamer in a circle using large arm movements. This action may be performed in front of or to the side of the body.
- *Small circles.* Using small arm movements, quickly make small circles to cause the streamer to look like a tornado.
- *Lasso.* Make large circles overhead.
- *Figure eights.* Move the arm so that it appears to be writing the number eight. This number eight will appear to have fallen over.
- *Windshield wipers.* Move the arm from side to side by starting down near the left hip, raising the arm overhead, and ending near the right hip. Repeat the action going from right hip to left hip.
- *Lion tamers.* Raise the streamer or rod overhead in front of the body, and then quickly snap it straight down to resemble the action of a lion tamer cracking a whip at a lion.
- *Running with the streamer.* Students love to run around the gym with the streamer trailing behind them as they run. They may carry it high or low. They also enjoy turning around in circles with the ribbon streaming around them.

You can use these ideas alone or combine them. The students may also be able to invent some new actions for the streamers.

HOCKEY PUCKS, STICKS, AND GOALS

Empty plastic containers from a popular item called Bubble Tape make perfect hockey pucks. Most students will be familiar with this product and should be able to provide an ample supply of empty containers in an amazingly short period of time. The only work involved is to remove the label, but that is not really necessary.

You can make very simple hockey sticks by using empty two-liter bottles. Again, no special work, except removing the labels (if desired), is required. For taller students, some bottled water products are packaged in taller plastic bottles. The students hold on to the neck of the bottle and try to hit the puck with the bottom of the bottle. You can construct a funnier version of a hockey stick by using a cardboard tube, the type in which posters often arrive, and a baby shoe. Stuff the tube into the opening of a shoe, approximately size three or four, and tie the laces. If the tube is not secure, you can attach it to the shoe using a glue gun. The students will have a fantastic time playing hockey with sticks that resemble little legs (see figure 1.2).

Expensive goals are not necessary when playing hockey. You can place two cones or area markers at the end of the playing area. If the puck goes between the markers, a goal is scored. Another idea is to cut two large boxes, such as the ones that are used to package refrigerators, to resemble goals.

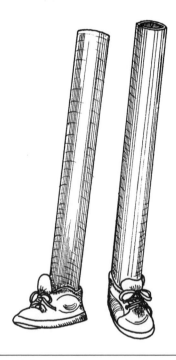

Figure 1.2 Hockey sticks

PINNIES

Pinnies are the jerseys that are worn over clothes so that teams can obviously be distinguished. (The old "shirts versus skins" method is no longer acceptable now that most schools have coed physical education classes.) You can make these pinnies with old towels. Fold the towel in half lengthwise and cut a half-moon neckline out of the towel. The neckline will need to be hemmed under or cut with pinking shears so that it will not fray. The children may simply put them on and wear them, or you can sew ribbon ties onto the sides of the towels for the children to tie them on. Cords may also be used as belts, if desired. Numbers may be sewn onto the pinnies if desired. If only two teams are used, the towels do not need to match. The teams would just be named the towels and the shirts. (Or the beach bunnies and the stuffed shirts, if you want to be more creative.) Smaller teams could try to match towel colors.

FOOTBALL T-STANDS

You can create a classy set of football tees from a single heavy-duty cardboard tube. Cut the tube into sections approximately two and a half inches long. Figure 1.3 illustrates how the cardboard circle that is left will hold a football on end so that the students can take a running kick at the football without another student having to hold it upright. If you do not have access to a band saw, you can use a hand saw to cut the tube; however, this is a time when an industrial arts teacher may be able to assist in the construction of equipment. Cutting the tube would be great practice for industrial arts students.

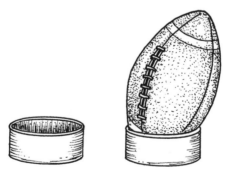

Figure 1.3   Football t-stands

BASES

Many activities, including baseball and a variety of tag games, require bases. Burlap sacks make terrific bases. The sacks can be filled with sawdust (the industrial arts teacher will be happy to accommodate this request), pine straw, old rags, or any other soft material. Fold over the sacks and place them on the field. When you are through with the bases, you can empty the sacks and save them to use for other purposes.

You can make permanent bases from old towels, canvas, or other heavy cloth. These items can be stitched together and filled with rags, panty hose, cotton, pine straw, or other appropriate material. Old carpet sample squares also make great bases. When they have become worn out from use in the gym, do not discard them. Save them to take outside for bases. Do not use bricks, rocks, or whole old tires as bases. They are dangerous, as students may trip on them and injure themselves. An old tire may be cut to use for a base if it is not a steel-belted tire.

WHISTLE HOLDER

You can make a handy whistle holder by using a shower curtain ring. Simply hook the shower curtain ring to the whistle (see figure 1.4) and then hook the ring onto a belt loop when the whistle is not being used. This holder keeps the whistle handy, and keeps it from flopping around the neck during running or other activity.

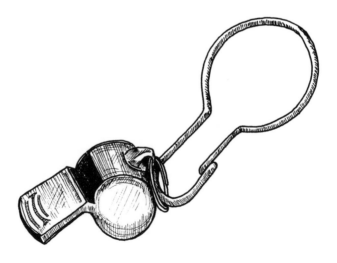

Figure 1.4   Whistle holder

TIME-OUT TIMER

Time-out is a common discipline procedure in physical education classes. Students who have been placed in time-out can be overlooked with all of the hustle and bustle of activity in the gym and may be left in time-out for a longer period than the teacher intended. Using the pendulum principle, you can make a simple timing device. You will need a #4 fishing sinker and some twine. Hang the sinker from a hurdle, a pull-up bar, the basketball goal, or any other item where the string attached to the sinker could be tied. The length of the twine is determined by the object to which it is tied. A pendulum string attached to the basketball goal would need to be considerably longer than one attached to the back of a chair.

The teacher swings the sinker, and when the sinker comes to a complete stop, the student is allowed to rejoin the group. The teacher determines the length of time spent in time-out by the strength put into the swing. The more severe the action resulting in time-out, the harder the pendulum is swung. The student should not sit near the pendulum as he or she may stop the swinging motion. When the pendulum comes to a complete stop, the student reports to the teacher, who verifies the stop, and then sends the student back into the class. Another simple means of timing a student in time-out is to take an old egg-timer from a board game that has lost some of its pieces and use it for timing a student. Games such as these may be found for a minimal cost at yard sales or the Salvation Army retail store.

CHAPTER 2

FROM TRASH TO TREASURE

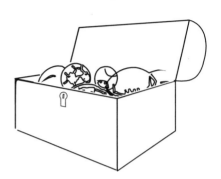

L ots of items that may have been previously discarded make wonderful additions to the physical education storeroom for new and exciting games. Most items may instantly be used in the gym without adapting them in any way. With a little creative thinking, former trash can be transformed into treasure! The reduce, reuse, recycle philosophy can go a long way toward enhancing the physical education possibilities and expanding the equipment inventory. After reading this chapter, you'll see trash in a whole new light.

OLD PANTY HOSE

Old panty hose have an endless number of possibilities when combined with a little creative thinking. Because a great number of educators are female, panty hose should be readily available in most schools. Merely placing a collection box in the faculty lounge will yield more panty hose than most physical educators can utilize.

Cutting the waist bands off the panty hose will provide you with your first resource. You can have the students place the bands around both feet and jump to a finish line. You can also use the bands to hold two students together for a variety of activities or games such as partner tag games or locomotor skills performed with a partner. Place the bands around the students' wrists or waists to hold the students together.

These bands are also excellent to use to shoot at targets. Place the band around the index finger and aim as if shooting a rubber band. Stretch the band with the other hand and fire by letting go. Other games can be played using this shooting concept.

HUNTER AND TARGET

This game is played with the panty hose waistbands being used as imitation bow and arrows. Each student is equipped with at least one band. The children are divided into groups of three or four students. One student is selected as the target. The target carries a wooden paint stirring stick with a paper plate or cardboard circle about the size of a paper plate attached to it. The other students, the hunters, attempt to hit the cardboard circle with their panty hose bands by pulling and letting go of the band, as if shooting a rubber band.

If the student misses the circle, he retrieves the band and tries again. If a student hits the circle, he replaces the target and gives a starting signal for the group to begin. The student posing as the target can pretend to be any animal he or she would like to be. This adds a little more excitement and creativity to the game.

WIGGLE WORMS

This game develops gross motor coordination and balance. A group of three or four students stands in a circle. There should be one panty hose waistband for each member of the group. On the starting signal, each person in the group must put the waistband over his or her head, wiggle his or her body through the band, and step out of the band. The band is then passed to the player on the right side of the wiggler. The next player must do the same thing. Because they are standing in a circle, they will continue to put one band after another over their heads and wiggle through them.

The game may continue for a specified amount of time or until the teacher gives a stopping signal. The groups may get a score, if desired, by adding up the number of times each member successfully completed wiggling through a band. If a player was halfway through the band when the stopping signal was given, that would not count as a completed point.

You can also use the legs of the old panty hose to make panty hose balls. To make the panty hose balls, cut off a leg of the old panty hose and then stuff the toe of the hose leg about three inches deep with batting, cotton, cut-up panty hose, or other soft material. Twist the leg of the panty hose three or four times close to the stuffing material. Then pull the leg back over the ball. Twist it again and pull the leg back over the ball one more time. Tie a knot in the panty hose as close to the ball as possible. Cut off any excess leg material that remains. Figure 2.1 illustrates the steps for making a panty hose ball. The result is a soft ball that has three layers of panty hose around the stuffing material.

Because panty hose come in a variety of colors, different groups may have different color balls so that they will be able to distinguish their balls when they go to retrieve them. You can use different color markers to put polka dots on the balls so students can tell them apart. Marking the balls this way can eliminate a lot of problems that arise

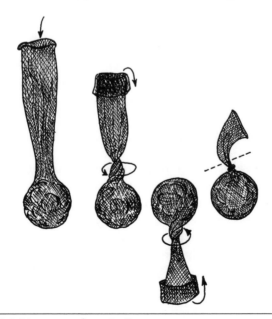

Figure 2.1   Making pantyhose balls

with younger children who become very possessive of the balls that are assigned to them. These balls are perfect for practicing throwing in a small area where students may get hit by balls. Many exciting games may also be played with these soft balls.

ROLY POLY BUGS

This game is excellent to play with younger children who are learning underhand throwing skills. The panty hose balls are very light and soft, making them easy to manipulate, and do not hurt when they contact the children. Divide the class into groups of two or four children. Then divide each of the groups into two teams and separate the teams by taping a line on the floor for each group.

One team starts as the throwers. Each thrower is given two or three panty hose balls. The other team must lie down on their backs on the other side of the dividing line. Without crossing the dividing line, the throwers try to hit the other team's players on the belly by using an underhand throw. If a player is hit in the belly, the player must curl up like a roly poly bug by bringing the knees up to the chest and holding onto them with the arms. As soon as each player has thrown all of his or her panty hose balls, the other team picks them up and becomes the throwers. Then the other team gets a turn to see how many roly poly bugs they can create.

MESSY BACKYARD

With this game, students can practice overhand throwing skills, underhand throwing skills, throwing with the nondominant hand, or kicking skills. You can use the game for all of the skills in one class period by changing the throwing method for each round of play. Set up the play area by dividing the floor with a dividing line and scattering the panty hose balls all over the floor, making sure each half of the floor has the same number of balls. Divide the class into two teams and tell each team that their half of the floor is their backyard. The object of the game is to clean up their backyard by throwing the mess (panty hose balls) out of their yard into the yard of the other team. Neither team is allowed to cross the dividing line that separates the two teams. At the end of two minutes, all students must "freeze" wherever they are, and the teacher will determine which team has the cleaner backyard.

SNOWBALL BATTLE

During the winter, you can use white panty hose balls for a snowball battle. The children will enjoy just throwing the snowballs at each other without any rules, or you can establish two teams with a dividing line between the teams. If the children begin to get bored, the rules that are outlined in the game Messy Backyard may be incorporated into the snowball battle.

SHOT IN THE FOOT

Each student is given one panty hose ball before the game starts. When the game begins, the students throw the panty hose balls and try to hit each other on the shoe without getting hit themselves. After the student throws the ball, he or she may pick up another ball from the floor, but a student may possess only one ball at a time. The students are free to go anywhere in the gym. The first time a student is hit by a ball, the student must hold one foot up and hop about the room to play. The second time a student is hit, the student must crawl around the room to play. The third time a student is hit, he or she must lay down on his or her belly. From this position, the student may continue to pick up a ball to throw and may move about to get the ball. When only one student or only a few students remain standing, the game is restarted with each player holding one ball.

OTHER USES

Panty hose legs are also useful for making rings. First cut off the foot, and then roll up the leg in a very tight roll. Tie the roll with yarn or other soft material in three or four places around the ring. You can use these rings for tossing to each other or for throwing at targets, but they are especially useful for children who have trouble seeing things. You can tie a bell to the ring so that the children can tell where the rings are when they are in motion. You can also tie these rings together to form a soft ball for throwing and catching. Again, placing a bell inside of the ball will assist visually impaired children in knowing where the ball is located. If you tie a panty hose leg to the ball and tie the other end of the leg to a wheelchair, students who are limited to a wheelchair may retrieve the ball by pulling it back with the panty hose leg.

Another idea for using old panty hose legs is to make items known as fox tails. Place a tennis ball in the toe of the stocking. Tie a knot in the leg as close to the ball as possible, as shown in figure 2.2. To make the fox tail game, draw lines on the leg of the hose with a permanent marker. Between the lines, put a number. The highest number should be closest to the ball, and the numbers should decrease from there. The players hold the end of the fox tail and circle their arms backwards. The player releases the tail when the ball is on the way up. Whatever number the player is holding upon catching the fox tail is the number of points that is awarded to the player. No points are awarded if the player catches the tennis ball part of the fox tail. The object of the game is to get the most points by catching the fox tail as close to the ball as possible without catching the ball itself. Children also like to just wind the fox tail in a large circle, and then let it go to see how far they can throw it. This activity, however, takes a large area such as a ball field so that students do not get hit by the fox tails.

You can also make badminton racquets and signs from the legs of panty hose. In addition to a panty hose leg, each racquet (and sign) requires a coat hanger and some duct tape. Pull the body of the coat hanger so that it forms a shape of a diamond. Straighten out the hook of the coat hanger to form the basis of the handle. Pull the leg of the hose over the diamond until the toe of the panty hose is on the top of the diamond. Pull the leg all of the way down the coat hanger. Wrap the leg of the panty hose several times around the handle area to provide protection there. Wrap the handles several times with the duct tape to provide safety and security at the handle. Be sure to check the handle before each use to be sure that the ends of the coat hanger wire are not about to protrude. The extra layers of panty hose and duct tape should prevent this, but it is always a good idea to

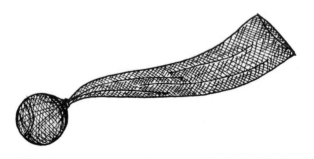

Figure 2.2   Fox Tails

check before using the racquets. You can transform these racquets into signs for activities, such as aerobic routines, by using markers or gluing felt shapes on the face of the racquet.

The only part of the panty hose that has not been utilized so far is the panty part. You can cut this part into strips to use for stuffing items such as panty hose balls, bases, or other items requiring a soft material for stuffing. You could use the entire panty hose for a tug-of-war rope for two small children. Each child would pull on one of the legs, trying to pull the panty part across the line to win.

Panty hose are one of the most versatile pieces of "trash" you can find. Their elasticity lends itself to a variety of purposes, and the various colors in which they are manufactured also allow for some creative inventions for physical education. Once a physical educator begins to use these items in the gym, the possibilities are limited only by the imagination.

OLD SOCKS

Socks should be sold in sets of three instead of pairs because it seems that one always disappears, leaving the other to sit alone for eternity. It would be difficult to find a house in the United States that did not have a set of old, unmatched socks laying around somewhere. Most people would be more than willing to donate these forlorn items to any physical education teacher that requested them. Of course, shortly after the socks were donated, most of the mates would show up under a bed or caught in the lint trap, but then there would be another set to be donated.

Old socks, like old panty hose, can make great stuffing material when a soft material is called for. You can make them into sock balls by stuffing the toe of the sock with one or two socks and then tying a knot in the sock as near to the stuffing as possible. You can fold excess material back over the ball or cut off the material. You can use these balls the same way you would use bean bags or panty hose balls. If you use a plastic bat, you can even use them to play baseball.

To make sock rockets for throwing and catching, follow the instructions for fox tails on page 18. Old socks may be tied together and used for blindfolds in any games requiring blindfolds. Use socks as temporary knee pads when playing games that require crawling by tying them around the backs of the legs. To keep together during a game, partners could each hold on to one end of the same sock instead of holding hands. If the socks have matches (they may have been donated due to holes in them), they can make an excellent method of pairing up students. Each student pulls a sock out of a box. The students are then paired together by finding the person who has the matching sock. The following games demonstrate just a fraction of the ways you can use old socks in physical education.

TURKEY TAILS

This super holiday game employs old socks. You can change the name of the game to Rabbit Tails, Reindeer Tails, Leprechaun Tails, or Cat Tails to fit the holiday. Students place approximately two inches of an old sock in their back pockets or in the waistband of their pants to make a tail. They are given approximately 45 seconds to run around the room gathering as many tails as possible from other students while trying not to lose their own tails. If players lose their tails, they may still run around pulling other tails. When time is up, students count the number of tails they have gathered and then return them to the other players. This game is usually good for about 10 minutes before the students become tired of it.

HIDE AND SOCK

This game is a great one to play outdoors, and it keeps the students running. One group of students hides the socks, and then the other half of the class looks for the socks. The teacher times the group to see how long it takes them to find all of the socks. When all of the socks have been found, the seeking group gets a turn to hide the socks. Then the other group gets a turn to look for the socks while the teacher times them. This game is fun to play around Easter when the students are excited about seeking games.

To ensure that students are not sitting idle during this game, the playing area may be divided into two sections by cones. Both groups hide socks at the same time, then both look for the socks that the other group has hidden at the same time. Both groups should have an equal number of socks. To keep the students moving quickly during the hiding phase, set a time limit for hiding the socks. If the socks have not been hidden by the end of the time limit, the students just drop them wherever they are standing when the signal is given to stop hiding socks.

MYSTERY SOCKS

Most any child will love this game. The mystery is intriguing for them, and the guessing part is fun. Put a small object inside of a sock and tie the sock. Prepare at least 15 socks with different objects inside each one. Some suggested objects to place inside the socks are a stopwatch, a spoon, a battery, a feather, a crayon, a penny, a rabbit's foot, a straw, a comb, a clothespin, a marble, a bar of soap, a plastic coin holder, an eraser, a pack of gum, a pacifier, a die, or a tape measure. Any object that is small and is not sharp would be appropriate. Put numbers all around the room, and then place a sock under each number. Older children can record on paper their guesses for what is in each sock. Younger children will just enjoy feeling the socks and trying to guess what is inside. After a specified period of time, approximately one minute per sock, meet in the middle of the gym and reveal what was in each sock. Do not open the socks, as this would cause an organizational problem for setting up the stations before the next class begins.

OLD NEWSPAPERS

Old newspapers are easily accessible and are fun to play with. One of the easiest items to construct with newspapers is newspaper balls. Making newspaper balls is a great job for students who cannot participate in physical education for some reason. While they are sitting out, they can crumple up sheets of newspapers into balls. You can use the newspaper balls to play Messy Backyard or Snowball Battle (see the rules for these games under the "Old Panty Hose" section).

You can roll up the newspapers to make even more useful items for the gym. Tape the rolls closed to use as relay batons for relay races or to throw for distance as in a javelin throw. The following games show some other ways you can use old newspapers in the gym.

PYRAMID

This game involves newspaper balls. The balls may already be constructed, or making the balls can be part of the game. Divide the students into groups of three or four. Give the groups five minutes to build the highest tower they can from newspaper balls. At the end of the five minutes, all students must step away from their pyramids to determine which is the tallest. The pyramid must be free-standing;

no one can help hold the paper. After the tallest pyramid is determined, the students are free to jump on their pyramids of newspaper balls as they would jump on piles of raked leaves.

CONSTRUCTION CREW (AND DEMOLITION TEAM)

This game is designed to develop teamwork and cooperative effort. This game is similar to Pyramid, except each group of two or three students is given a stack of flat newspapers. The groups must construct an original tower or building out of the papers. The papers may be rolled, wadded, or folded in any method that the group desires. Consider allowing the students to use scotch tape. Give the groups between five and ten minutes to design and construct an original piece of architecture. The building should be judged on creativity. If desired, you can give a title to each group's structure, such as most creative, most unusual, tallest, widest, wildest, most realistic, looks most like an animal, or any other creative title you come up with. After the pieces of architecture have been created and viewed, the students will turn into the demolition team to destroy the building. This activity will be as much, or possibly more, fun than building and designing the structure. Each group should be responsible for the cleaning up of the materials that it used for construction.

SPEED CLEAN

Cleaning up the old newspapers after they have been used for a game can be a game in itself. Have a race to see which group can clean up its own area first. Another version of this clean-up game that is usually successful is to give each group a large trash bag and allow the students to pick up any old newspapers that are in the room, even if they were not used by their group. On the starting signal, the students pick up as much of the mess as they can without running into each other. Running into someone results in a penalty of dumping whatever is in the runner's hands into the bag of the person who was run into. The group that has the heaviest trash bag when the clean-up is finished wins the game.

BEAT THE CLOCK

In this clean-up game, you time the first class to do the clean-up to see how long it takes them to clean up the mess that the class made. Their time and the date, along with the name and grade of their class, are posted as the record time on a poster in the gym. Whenever a class beats the record, the old time and date are crossed out, and the new class time and date are posted.

COSTUME PARTY

This game is yet another variation of Pyramid and Construction Crew where teamwork and cooperative effort are necessary for the group to be successful. This game would fit nicely in a unit of cooperative games. In this game, the students use the newspapers to make a costume for one of the members of the group. They may dress up the member to resemble a sports figure, a famous person, a historical character, a cartoon character, or an animal. They may roll, wad, fold, or punch holes through the newspapers to design the costumes.

At the end of a specified time period, the people in the costumes may either stand still while the rest of the class moves around to view them, or they may parade down a make-believe runway. The class will gather around the runway to view the characters in their costumes. When this game is completed, the models go to several students who have been assigned as dressing-room attendants. These students have a large trash bag into which the models can drop their costumes as they remove them.

PAPER CHASE

In this fast-paced activity, students place a quarter of a sheet of newspaper, approximately 10 x 14 inches, on their chests. They remove their hands from the paper and must move about the room quickly enough for the paper to stay on their chests. You can use this activity as a warm-up or make it into a more complicated game by adding a few rules. The rules could be that any students who drop their sheets must do a specified stunt before they are allowed to get back up. Stunts could include log rolling across the room, walking 20 steps like a duck, crawling across the room with the newspaper on their heads, laying down on their backs with their hands and feet in the air until they finish singing the alphabet song, or wiggling across the room on their bellies like a snake. You could make this activity into a game where the students who drop their papers must crawl on the floor with their papers on their backs until only one student is left standing. The last student who is standing would be the winner of the round. Then all of the crawling students would stand up, and you could replace crawling with a different locomotor skill.

EQUESTRIAN RACE

Roll up newspapers lengthwise and use them for the horses in an equestrian race. Each horse has three riders that ride at the same time. All three of the riders straddle the newspaper and must run to a designated spot or run a designated number of laps around the room while riding the horse. To make the race more difficult, one or two of the players can face backward as they race. If any of the players are facing backward, the race should be turned into a walking race rather than a running race. This race will also work with two riders if the riders are too big to fit three onto a horse.

SOCCER SNATCH

Each student wads a sheet of newspaper into a tight ball and places it on the floor in front of him or her. The newspaper has now become a soccer ball. The soccer ball can only be moved by controlled kicking. As the students are kicking their soccer balls throughout the gym, the teacher moves about saying, "I am the Soccer Snatcher and I snatch soccer balls!" The teacher tries to snatch the soccer balls away from the students as they kick them throughout the gym. If the teacher does manage to snatch a soccer ball from one of the students, the student must walk backwards for five giant steps where the teacher will kick the ball back to the student to continue practicing controlled kicking and dodging the teacher.

For a variation with older students, select several students to be the snatchers. The snatchers do not have a soccer ball when the game begins. If a snatcher stops another player's soccer ball with one of his or her feet, the snatcher gets to keep the soccer ball. The student who loses a soccer ball becomes a snatcher and must try to snatch another student's soccer ball. No students are ever eliminated, and the students are constantly moving.

HAPPY HATS

This game can be used for younger children while practicing basic locomotor skills such as walking, running, hopping, jumping, skipping, or galloping. Students place the newspapers on their heads with the crease for the page on the top of their heads, like hats.

Everyone performs the designated locomotor skill throughout the gym while trying to keep the newspaper on top of their heads. If the hat falls off, the student must stop where the hat falls off and ask the closest student for help. This student helps by bending down, trying not to lose her own hat, picking up the fallen hat, and placing it on the bare head of the student who had lost the hat. Once a child has been helped, he thanks the kind helper, and both students continue with the locomotor skill in progress.

Once your newspapers have outlived their usefulness for your physical education classes, don't discard them as trash. They can go into a recycling bin or be donated to a pet shelter or humane society that can use them in animals' cages. Many of the animals prefer these papers as they are already used, therefore providing them with something interesting to smell while they are confined to their cages!

OLD SODA BOTTLES

You can use the smaller, 16-ounce plastic soda bottles to make bowling pins. Put a little sand or water in the bottom of each bottle to give it a little stability. The students may use these pins for regular bowling just using a playground ball for a bowling ball. They can also be used for obstacles in relay races or for obstacles to weave around when learning to control a soccer ball. In addition, they can be used in an obstacle course for jumping over in various ways. For instance, students would have to jump green bottles by using a straddle jump and jump clear bottles by using a tuck jump. You can also incorporate soda bottle pins into games.

PIN RACE

This active game helps students get their heart rate up and develop some aerobic endurance. Divide the class into two teams. Use about 30 bottles for each team, but each team should have different colors. Green and clear plastic bottles are probably the easiest to find. There should be twice as many bottles for each team as there are players to ensure that no students are idle during the game. Set a time period, such as two minutes. In that two minutes, the teams try to knock over all of the other team's bottles. The teams are also allowed to put up any of their own bottles that they find knocked over. No one may knock over or pick up the same bottle two times in a row; the player must move on to a different bottle after touching a bottle. At the end of a specified time limit, all players must sit down while the leader decides which team has the most bottles left standing.

The game will be more exciting if each round adds a new challenge. The challenges could include knocking the bottles over with the elbows, knocking the bottles over with the knees, moving through the room doing the crab walk, picking the bottles up with the elbows, keeping hands behind the back at all times, or using the duck walk to move through the room. Another variation is having two members of the same team connected to each other as they play by holding hands, locking elbows, or each holding on to the end of a sock. Then change partners so that one player from the green team is connected in the same manner to one player on the clear team.

HUMAN BOWLING BALLS

This game is great to play when teaching tumbling. The students are required to tumble and become aware of the amount of space that they require to do a series of rolls. Divide the class into groups of two students so that there are no long waits between turns. Toward the end of a mat or two connected mats, set up plastic soda bottles in a triangle to resemble a set of bowling pins. It may be helpful to put masking tape on the mat where each of the bottles is to be placed so that the students can replace the bottles for each other as they finish their turns. The object of the game is for the students to roll like bowling balls so that they knock down the bottles.

The students face the bottles, find a starting place on the mat, and do forward rolls toward the bottles. If using a single mat, they are allowed two forward rolls toward the pins (they must do two, but are not allowed to do three.) If using two connected mats or a longer single mat, the students may be required to do three or four rolls before stopping. This will be a little more fun as they may find that it is difficult to roll straight when rolling several rolls without stopping. If students do not get all the way to the pins in the allotted number of rolls, it is considered a gutter ball and no score is given. If they do reach the pins and knock them down, one point is given for each pin knocked down. No special formulas for strikes are given; strikes simply count for 10 points.

Blindfolded Bowling is a more complicated version of this game that you can use for older students. The game is the same except that the person rolling wears a blindfold. The students in the group can coach the student with verbal cues, but the student is not allowed to stop rolling.

PACKING PEANUTS

Generally thought of as a nuisance and a landfill waste, packing peanuts can be a super item to have in the physical education storage room. Be sure that the peanuts are not the new kind that disintegrate when wet. Although these peanuts, which are made of starch, are an incredible breakthrough for the environment, they are not nearly as sturdy as the Styrofoam ones, and they will disappear if they come in contact with any water. This could be a potential problem in an old gym that has leaks or one with skylights that tend to leak whenever it rains. Styrofoam peanuts lend themselves to many different types of activities.

PEANUT PUSH

This game develops hand-eye coordination and locomotor skills. It also makes an appropriate field day activity. This game can be played in several ways. Players could push the peanuts to a finish line with their noses. Because the packing peanuts are so light, you could change this activity to have the players blow the peanuts to the finish line or marker. Another variation is to have the players use a plastic baseball bat or empty plastic soda bottle to push the peanut across the floor.

STREET SWEEPER

This game requires an old broom for each team of two or three children and lots of packing peanuts. The peanuts are scattered throughout the gym. Each team tries to sweep up the biggest pile of peanuts. One person from each group runs out and sweeps as many peanuts to his or her team as possible. As soon as each student returns to their team, the next student from each team runs out and sweeps back more peanuts to add to his or here team's pile. This continues until all of the peanuts have been swept off the floor.

NEEDLE IN A HAYSTACK

This activity is appropriate for a school carnival or for a field day. Fill a small plastic wading pool with packing peanuts. Hide some small objects, such as small dog treats that are shaped like bones, inside the peanuts. The students have 30 seconds to see how many bones they can find. If they find five or more, they receive a small prize. You could also hide candy in the packing peanuts. After 30 seconds, or once the student has found two or three pieces of candy, the next student in line has a turn to search.

OLD COFFEE CANS

Old coffee cans make great storage containers for small objects, such as clothespins or table tennis balls, because they can be sealed, thereby preventing a disaster if a can is knocked off of a storage shelf. In addition, coffee cans can also be incorporated as equipment in a physical education program, such as playing pieces for games. To prevent accidents or cuts, be sure there are no rough edges to the coffee cans prior to using them as game pieces. Also, do not throw away the can lids; they make excellent Frisbees.

Coffee Can Races are a fresh and different way to practice soccer skills and foot-eye or hand-eye coordination. To do this activity, use the cans with their lids on them to eliminate the possibility of students coming into contact with any rough edges of the cans. Put the cans on their sides and have the students roll them with their feet. The students can also use a stick or a bat to roll the cans along the floor.

OLD DRYER SHEETS

Juggling is an excellent hand-eye coordination activity to teach to children, but often the cost of juggling scarves prohibits the physical educator from being able to incorporate juggling into the curriculum. If double classes are taught, then often the cost of the scarves would equal at least half, if not more, of the entire physical education budget for the year. Most physical educators cannot justify spending half of their budgets on equipment that is limited to a single activity. An alternative to juggling scarves is old dryer sheets.

The sheets must have been through the dryer at least once, though, or they will be too stiff to use. If they have been through the dryer more than once, they will soften a little more and will float in the air a little longer. The dryer sheets do not float quite as long as juggling scarves, and they are not nearly as colorful, but they certainly are cost-effective. They are also much easier to use for learning to juggle than tennis balls or Indian clubs. Additionally, they do not stray from the juggler when dropped like balls do; therefore, students are more easily contained in a small area. The students will be pleased with the success they will achieve with the dryer sheets.

M & M MINIS PLASTIC TUBE CONTAINERS

M & M Minis are packaged in a sturdy plastic tube that has a flip top on it. They come in several colors, including green, blue, yellow, red, and orange. The lids are attached to the tube by a plastic piece, so they are not easily lost. The sturdy plastic makes them a durable piece of equipment for playing games.

A game called the Tube Tower Race game may be played once you have collected five tubes of each color. Each team, consisting of two or three players, is assigned a color that coordinates with the colors of the tubes. The tubes are scattered throughout the gym. The first person on a team must go out in the gym and find a tube to match the team's color. That student brings it back to the group and sets it on the floor in front of the group. The next member of the team must find another tube of the same color and bring it back, stacking it on top of the first tube. The next player cannot go get another tube until the tower can balance by itself. This process continues with players going to get another tube until all of a team's tubes have been gathered and are in a free-standing tower. A variation of this game would be to have each member of the team bring back a different color. If a member got back to the team to find that the color brought back was already in the tower, he or she would have to return that tube to the floor and pick up another tube for the tower. When completed, each tower would have five different colors in it.

EMPTY ADDING MACHINE PAPER ROLLS

When rolls of adding machine paper run out, you are left with sturdy plastic rolls that are about two and a half inches long. These rolls are usually white and can be saved until there are enough to make an interesting game. When approximately three rolls per student in the class have been accumulated, the Fossil Hunting game can be played.

To play this game, spread the white plastic rolls all over the gym floor. Tell the students that these are fossils and dinosaur bones; they should never be touched by human hands if they are found on a fossil-hunting excursion. Divide the students into several groups and give each group special fossil-hunting tools to recover the bones and fossils. These tools could be a plastic drinking straw, a dowel rod, a plastic baseball bat, a long glue stick for a glue gun, a pencil, or any other long instrument that can be used to push the roll back to the group's collection point.

The first student in the group hunts for a fossil, and when the student finds one, he or she rolls it back to the collection point for the group. If a student touches a fossil with his or her hands, he or she must return the fossil to its original site and go back to the group with no fossil. The group may use a hula hoop to keep the fossils in at their collection point. The group members lift the hoop for the hunter when the hunter rolls the fossil back. Then another student in the group goes out and looks for more fossils. This hunting continues until all of the bones have been recovered. The group that recovers the most bones and fossils wins the game.

GARDEN HOSE

You can make or adapt numerous items from garden hose. If the hose is fairly long, it can be used instead of rope for playing tug-of-war to eliminate the possibility of rope burns. You can also use the plastic hose to teach rope jumping skills to younger children. Because it does not twist, some children who are having trouble jumping a rope may find it easier to jump the hose. Other uses for plastic hose include jump rope handles, relay batons for track and field races, and markers to indicate boundaries or important lines in games. The hose may also be used to play the limbo by stretching it out between two players who act as the holders for that round as the others pass under.

EMPTY PAPER TOWEL ROLLS

Paper towel rolls are a useful item to have when teaching games that require cooperative skills. A group could use the rolls to build a log cabin. Using long rolls from paper towels and short rolls from toilet paper together can make a more interesting and more challenging log cabin. The group must design and build the log cabin together; all members of the group must participate. Give the group a time limit to build the cabin. When finished, the cabin must stand by itself.

CARDBOARD BOXES

You can use just about any size of box for a game. Students can stand inside shoe boxes as if they were skates. The students may perform any activity using these skates. They may run a race, play a game such as volleyball, or toss a Frisbee to each other. You can call these boxes cross-country skis and have the students run a race or go through an obstacle course on these skis. A larger box could be a bobsled or dogsled for the students. One student sits inside the box while two or three others push that student around the room. That student gets out of the box and another rider gets in until all have had a turn to be pushed around the room while inside the box.

A medium box may be used to run a version of a three-legged race. Two students standing side-by-side place the inside foot inside the box. They must work together to move across the floor. A sturdy medium box may make a great table.

You can use large boxes as tunnels for obstacle courses. Cut the top and the bottom out of the box and place it on its side. If the box seems as though it might fall over, place a chair on both sides of the box with the back of the chair against the box. The chairs should give the box the stability it was missing. If the box is quite long, more than one chair may be necessary for each side. Also, teachers have been known to make desks and file folder containers out of larger boxes.

Another use for cardboard boxes is the Speedy Marble game. This game develops fine motor skills and hand-eye coordination. This game is played with two players. You could set up several stations in the gym with two people playing at each. The two players face each other with a small, flat box between them. Inside the box is approximately 50 marbles. Two cans or small shoe boxes without lids are placed on each side of the box containing the marbles. The two containers that are nearest the player are the ones that the player uses. See figure 2.3.

When the observing player calls "Go!," the two players pick up two marbles at a time, one in each hand. They drop them into the shoe boxes or cans that are outside the box. The players should not stop if a marble does not land inside. When all of the marbles are gone, the one that has the most marbles in his or her shoe box or can is considered the winner. After a few minutes, the students may be given a signal to stop so that they may change partners.

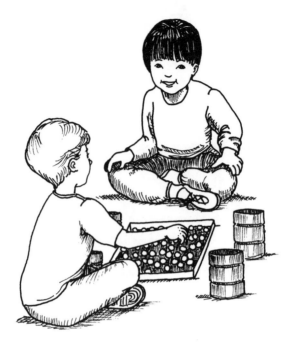

Figure 2.3   Speedy Marble game formation

PLASTIC TRASH BAGS

A wonderful activity to do in the spring to celebrate Earth Day uses trash bags. This active, running game is a great method of aerobic exercise. Groups of students are given a bag and are informed of the time limit. They then proceed to search the school campus, picking up any litter that they may find. The entire school could participate in this activity simultaneously. The group that finds the most litter within the specified time period reigns over any other Earth Day festivities that should occur that day. All the children could parade to the dumpster with the trash bags with the group that had the most trash leading the parade.

CHAPTER 3

SAME OLD STUFF

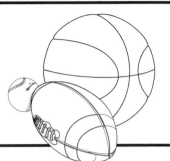

This chapter will explore creative and innovative methods of reviving the same old equipment. It will demonstrate methods of using traditional equipment in nontraditional ways. Finding new uses for existing equipment stretches your physical education budget with delightful results. The students will be excited about the new activities, and the physical education department won't have any additional costs.

FRISBEES

With a little creativity, Frisbees can be versatile pieces of equipment. They may be used for playing some thrilling games or incorporated into the main piece of equipment for an entire series of relay races. An entire class period can be consumed with Frisbee games and activities. These games and activities may include the following:

1. Jump with the Frisbee between the knees.
2. Hold the Frisbee between the elbows while running.
3. Hold the Frisbee with two hands behind the back while running.
4. Hold the Frisbee against the chest using the chin and walk or run, keeping the Frisbee against the chest.
5. Balance the Frisbee on the head while walking.
6. Balance the Frisbee on one hand like a waiter carrying a tray while walking.
7. Balance the Frisbee on the stomach while doing the crab walk.
8. Use two Frisbees upside down to put the feet in while sliding down the floor.
9. Run using the Frisbee as a steering wheel.
10. Two people must put the Frisbee between them and carry it without touching it with the hands.
11. Two people run holding the Frisbee; one person holds it with two hands behind the back, and the other person holds it with two hands in front. Both are facing forward.
12. Two people go as fast as possible holding the Frisbee. Both hold it with two hands behind the back. One person faces forward while the other person faces backward.
13. Two people hold the Frisbee between their backs, not touching it with the hands. They walk while one faces forward and the other faces backward.
14. The entire group gathers around the Frisbee, holding onto it with one hand. They must cooperatively move to the goal and back.

Frisbees are quite cost-effective when they are used in several games instead of just being tossed around on occasion. The following games are just a sampling of the possibilities.

STAR WARS

This game moves fast, and the players do plenty of sprinting. This game is also intended for students who are in the fourth grade or higher. Divide the students into four equal teams with only three or four players in a team. There may be two or three sets of games going simultaneously.

Seat the students in teams along the four lines of a square. Each student in the group is numbered from one to the number of members in each team. There should be four players with each number, one from each of the four different teams. In front of each team, in the center of the square, is a Frisbee with a bean bag in it, as seen in figure 3.1. When the teacher says a number, the students from each team with that number must get the beanbag out of the Frisbee, go out of the space where he or she started, and then run around behind each of the team members counterclockwise. He or she then returns through the space where he or she left to run and replaces the bean bag into the Frisbee. The first one back from the race around the team scores a point for the team. Let the children pretend the bean bags are planets they are racing around the universe trying to save. Thus, the name "Star Wars."

The bean bag must be completely inside the Frisbee before a team can be considered finished. If a player throws the bean bag at the Frisbee, but it does not go in, that player must go after the bean bag to put it in the Frisbee. To add some variation, the students may be in a push up position, doing curls, stretching a straddle stretch, or performing other athletic stunts while waiting for their number to be called.

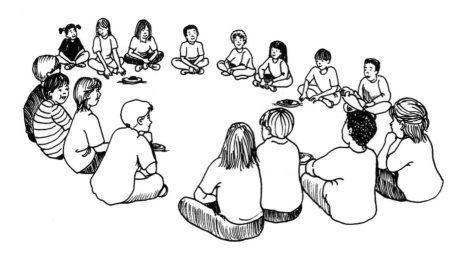

Figure 3.1   Star Wars formation

CROSS THE RIVER

This cooperative game uses one more Frisbee for each group than members of the group. All members of the group must be connected in one way or another. Each student must touch the student in front of him or her on the shoulder or arm to remain connected. The students must go from one side of the room to the other side of the room using the Frisbees. The first player in the group puts a Frisbee down and steps into it. The players in the line pass another Frisbee to the first player who puts it down and moves onto it. All players must move by placing their feet in the Frisbees. They may have to share a Frisbee with another player when they each have one foot inside a Frisbee. The group moves along as the last player keeps passing the last Frisbee on the floor up the line to the first player who puts it down and steps into it (see figure 3.2). Each player moves up another Frisbee and the last player passes the last Frisbee up the line again. This process continues until all players have crossed the room.

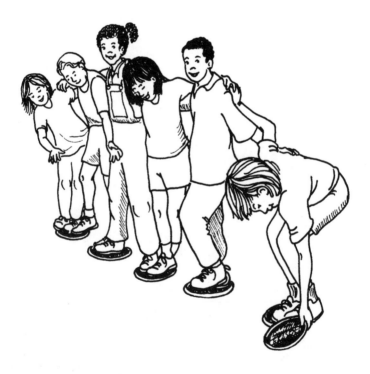

Figure 3.2 Cross the River

FRISBEE GOLF

This game is similar to golf in the fact that the lower the score, the better the game the player has played. Several holes should be set up for the players to attempt. There should be enough holes that two or three players would be the most assigned to a group and all groups would be able to participate simultaneously. This game requires a large playing area such as a baseball or football field. If the class is large, the players may not get to play every hole on the first day.

Each player has a Frisbee and tries to hit a goal at each station or hole. Goals may be knocking over an aluminum can that is sitting on a milk carton, putting the Frisbee through a hula hoop that is hanging from a tree, or getting it into a box. These goals should be adapted to the environment in which the students will be playing. The students travel in groups of two or three. One of them may be assigned to keep score for the group, or each individual may be charged with keeping his/her own score. The students count the number of throws it takes to accomplish the task that is assigned at each hole. Each hole should have a specific throwing point from which the Frisbee must always be thrown. A maximum of five throws per hole should be allowed. If a student has not made the assigned goal after five throws, the student should record a score of six for that hole and proceed with the group to the next hole. At the conclusion of the entire course, the students should total their scores for all of the holes so the teacher can average them to see what the "par for the course," should be.

FRISBEE BASEBALL

This game is very much like baseball, except a Frisbee is substituted for the bat and ball. The field is set up with bases as in baseball, and the fielding team may place a player on each of the bases, in the shortstop position, on the catcher's mound, and at the home plate. The "batter" throws the Frisbee to the outfield, or the "batter" may drop the Frisbee in front of the home plate for a bunt. The batter then runs for first base. The fielders must tag the batter with the Frisbee to get him or her out, unless it is a forced run. In the case of a forced run, the fielders need only to tag the base where the runner is headed to get the runner out. After three outs, the teams switch places. A point is scored whenever a runner makes it back to the home plate without being tagged out. A variation of this game is to let all players on the batting team have a turn before the teams switch places.

FRISBEE JUGGLING

This game is played with five players and four Frisbees per group. The students stand in the formation of a star. The players throw the Frisbee to the same person every time, making a pattern of a star as they throw. Have the students practice throwing in the proper order for a few minutes before adding more Frisbees. After the students have accomplished the pattern, add one Frisbee at a time. The students continue to follow the throwing pattern with two Frisbees, then three, and finally four Frisbees being thrown through the group at the same time, as illustrated in figure 3.3.

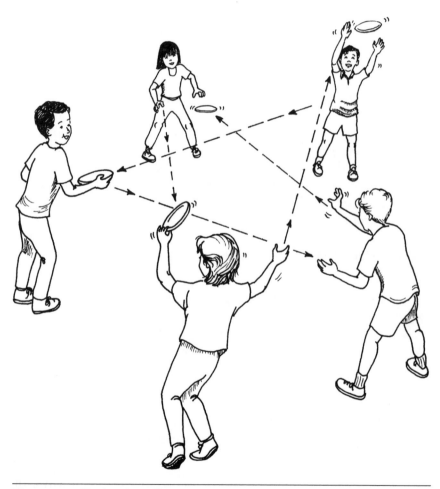

Figure 3.3   Frisbee Juggling

RUBBER GLOVES

In these days of infectious diseases, all schools have latex gloves readily available. You can inflate a glove like a balloon and use it as an unusual sort of ball. The students can play volleyball with the inflated glove over a net. If you can acquire enough gloves, the students may play the game in pairs. With pairs, a net is optional. The students may merely volley the glove between themselves trying to see how many volleys they can do without the glove touching the floor.

A variation of this activity is to divide the students into small groups and have each group stand in a circle with one student in the middle. The middle person should be allowed to stay in the middle for two rounds before a new person moves to the middle. A round consists of as many volleys as possible among the group. When the glove hits the ground, the round is ended.

JUMP ROPES

A creative way of incorporating jump ropes into an obstacle course is to lay them on the floor overlapping each other and call that area the "snake pit." The students must attempt to cross the snake pit without waking any of the snakes. If they step on a jump rope, or snake, they will awaken the snake and most likely receive a snake bite. They must carefully tiptoe through the snake pit. You could also hang the ropes from a basketball goal and have the students try to go between the rope snakes without touching them.

STILTS

A favorite item of children of all ages is stilts. If your school has purchased stilts, sometimes called tom walkers, they probably sit in the physical education storeroom until field day. You can use these idle stilts in many activities.

FOLLOW THE LEADER

The students take turns leading a line of three or four students through a designated area by creatively moving on the stilts. These creative movements may include walking forward, sideways, or backward; marching; high stepping with straight legs; stepping with giant steps; bending the knees so that the feet rise near the bottom; or duck walking. After approximately 30 seconds to one minute, the leader goes to the end of the line, and the new leader takes over trying to move in new and different ways.

BALANCING CONTESTS

Students can challenge other students to balancing contests, or the teacher can hold a giant balancing contest for the group. While on stilts, students may attempt to stand on one foot (stilt) for a designated period of time. If the other foot (stilt) touches the ground, the student puts it back up and counts it as a touch. At the end of the time period, the students add up the number of touches they had. Then the other foot is held up for the same time period. Older students will be able to hold a foot up for longer periods than the younger students.

OBSTACLE COURSES

You can construct courses for the students involving going around, under, over, or through a variety of objects while they are on their stilts.

LINE DANCING

You could teach a simple line dance, such as the bunny hop or the conga, to the students and then have the students perform the dance on stilts. If the students are able to learn a more complicated line dance, they will have great fun performing it on stilts.

PARACHUTE

The parachute is an excellent piece of equipment for the development of the upper body, but it is also a versatile decorative item. You can use the parachute to help create the exciting atmosphere of the circus right in the gym (see figure 3.4). First, string the parachute with a rope through the hole in its center and tie the rope to a rafter on the ceiling. Then using string tied to the handles, pull the parachute out so that it resembles a circus tent. Attach the other ends of the strings to the walls in the gym or other stationary objects to provide tension on the parachute so that it keeps the shape of the circus tent. You can use this tent to set the stage for a challenging obstacle course based on circus themes. This is an amusing way to incorporate motor skills into the daily curriculum.

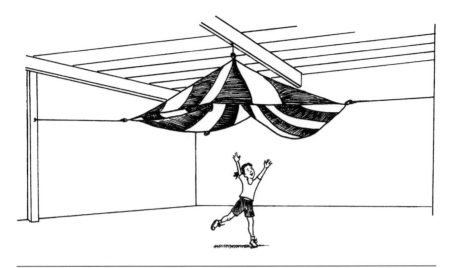

Figure 3.4   Circus tent

To cue the students as to what to do around the room, make signs from cardboard boxes or panty hose legs (p.18). Draw pictures of animals or circus-related things or cut the pictures out of magazines and place them on the boxes. Just after the circus does come to town, ask merchants for the advertisement posters that have been hung in their stores. Most will be grateful to have someone to remove the posters for them. Use these posters to decorate the hallway that leads to the gym. This decoration will create some curiosity and excitement before the students ever reach the gym. Any combination of the following circus activities will create a fun obstacle course to be performed under the colorful circus tent.

TIGHT ROPE

Have the students walk across the low balance beam. For circus appearances, they may be required to carry a piece of PVC pipe or a small umbrella. If no balance beam is available, lay a long piece of rope on the floor for the children to walk upon, and they may pretend it is in the air.

ACROBATS

The students can do forward rolls or log rolls across a mat to imitate circus acrobats. At the end of the mat, the students should stand with their hands in the air and say a loud, "Tah Dah!"

CLOWNS

This station will definitely be a hit with children. Put a variety of equipment at this station, such as large and small balls, jump ropes, stuffed animals, large shoes, or hula hoops, and tell the students they have to create something silly before they can continue to the next station. The students will love being able to be a clown without getting in trouble, and most will be able to use their imaginations to allow them to do something silly. Others may imitate something they saw another child do in that station. Some children may even display some cooperative skills and create some silly actions with another student.

JUGGLERS

Place juggling scarves or old dryer sheets in this area to give students an opportunity to try to juggle. This station will run more smoothly if the students have had some exposure to the techniques of juggling before they try it in the middle of an obstacle course.

ELEPHANTS

Have an area where the students do an elephant walk across the floor or around a circle.

TRICK DOGS

Put some hula hoops in this area. When two students arrive, one is the dog trainer, and the other can be the dog. The trainer holds the hoop up for the dog to jump through. Then the two partners trade places, and the trainer can have a turn at being the dog.

BEARS

In this station, mark a circle on the floor with masking tape, ropes, or paint. The students do the bear walk around this circle. It might be fun for the students to growl ferociously during this activity.

LIONS

The teacher should be in this station with a small chair, a rhythmic ribbon (bought or made), and a folded tumbling mat. The students are the lions and the teacher is the tamer. The teacher cracks the whip (the ribbon or a jump rope if a ribbon cannot be found or made) and the lion jumps on all fours onto the folded tumbling mat. When the lion tamer cracks the whip a second time, the lion jumps down from the mat and continues around the obstacle course. This station should be placed in the corner of the room so that the teacher may face the entire gym. The teacher can then supervise all of the activities while acting as the lion tamer.

SNAKE CHARMERS

The students can stop at this station to pretend they are cobras being charmed out of a basket. Then they should slither across the floor to the next station.

SIAMESE TWINS

When a student reaches this station, he or she must wait until the next student arrives so that they may be Siamese twins. The two students must place an item between them, such as a playground ball, a Frisbee, or a bean bag. They must then let go of the item with their hands and keep the item pressed between them while walking around the area set up for displaying the Siamese twins.

TRAPEZE ARTIST

Ideally, this station would have a bar for students to swing on. If no such bar is available, a climbing rope would also work. You could also hang a rope from the backboard of a basketball goal for the children to have an area to swing. If this activity is done outdoors, the monkey bar on a jungle gym would work. Any item where the students have an opportunity to swing themselves in any manner can be used to help students pretend that they are trapeze artists swinging through the air.

HORSEBACK RIDERS

An old saddle is perfect for this activity. Place the saddle on the floor or on top of a folding mat. The students, one at a time, try to balance while standing on the saddle. They pretend that they are standing on a real horse. If you don't have a saddle, you can use a balance board or anything that is a challenge to stand on. Old Pogo bounce balls would work if you can find them.

PLANK JUMPER

Find a small child's swimming pool that is made of hard plastic; don't use the inflatable kind. These pools are often discarded due to a crack which causes them to leak. Because no water will be put in the pool, it is acceptable if it has a leak. Fill the pool approximately two-thirds full of packing peanuts. Have some extra in a plastic bag in case they get compressed from this activity. Blue or green peanuts will look more realistic. The students jump from a plastic milk crate or from the end of a folded mat into the pool of packing peanuts.

SEALS

The students pretend that they are seals, and they attempt to balance a ball on their noses. Playground balls may be used for this activity if beach balls are not available.

THE STRONG PERSON

Inflate two balloons, black or brown ones if available, and attach one of them to each end of a PVC pipe or broomstick. For an additional visual effect, use a permanent marker to write *500 pounds* on each of the balloons. The students pretend that this "barbell" is very heavy as they perform a "clean and jerk" move with it.

FOLDING MATS

Folding mats may be used in a variety of ways in addition to tumbling. Think of them as building blocks. Folding mats can be stacked to resemble steps to enable small children to reach higher equipment. For instance, students may not be able to reach a chinning bar on the wall without the assistance of a teacher. Because the students can use the steps, the teacher is no longer required to be there to assist the students to reach the bar. You also can create a variety of obstacle course stations and other activities with folding mats.

BALL PIT

This activity is useful for developing gross motor coordination in small children. Place four folding mats at right angles to each other so that they form the outline of a square. Fill the open area with balls of any kind, as seen in figure 3.5. Playground balls are excellent fillers for the ball pit. If students fall from the mats into the pit, they bounce around on playground balls. The students also find it fun and challenging to wade through and to climb over the balls in the pit. This activity resembles the ball pits that are often found at playgrounds at fast food restaurants.

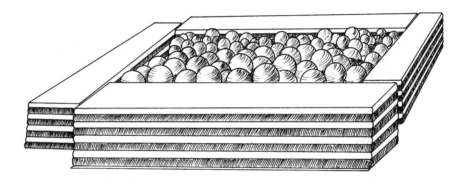

Figure 3.5   Folding mat ball pit

VAULT AND VAULTING BOARD

Often gymnastics equipment is beyond the budget of a school. Folding mats may be used to provide an opportunity for students to experience the activities and motor patterns that are used in gymnastics. To create a substitute for a vaulting horse, place two or three folding mats on top of each other while they are folded. The folded mats may be turned sideways for a vaulting horse or lengthwise for long-horse vaulting.

If a vaulting springboard is not available, place a folded tumbling mat in front of the "vaulting horse." The mat being used for the springboard should remain folded and be turned perpendicular to the vaulting horse. Tape a piece of masking tape, approximately 12 inches long, on the springboard mat to show the students where the feet need to be placed. This mark will be similar to a real springboard which has a line on it for the placement of the feet when vaulting. With this setup, students can learn the proper placement of the hands when vaulting, the proper method of using a springboard, and experience the feeling of vaulting over a horse as in gymnastics. To avoid possible accidents, the instructor should check the mats for slippage after each vaulter to be sure they are properly placed for the next student.

TUNNELS

Folding mats may be folded so that they may be used as tunnels in an obstacle course. Pull the mat up at one of the folds to create a triangle. As in figure 3.6, students can then crawl through this hole.

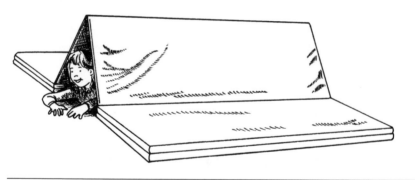

Figure 3.6   Folding mat tunnel

THE WORLD'S FATTEST BALANCE BEAM

If students are unable to experience the feeling of challenge that occurs when performing on a balance beam because the school does not own one, the students may still be challenged by creating a situation where they must be precise in their movements and tumbling or they could fall. This goal may be accomplished by using a folded tumbling mat or aligning two folded mats lengthwise to create a longer beam. Place open mats around the folded mat so students will land on an open mat if they fall off the created beam. Although this newly created beam is considerably wider than the four inches held by a real balance beam, the students still must align their movements such as rolls and cartwheels, or they will fall off the side of the folded mat.

Using a folded mat beam is certainly more challenging than performing the same move on the floor, but it is not nearly as challenging as trying the move on a real beam. A folded mat balance beam can be a superb transition for students working on learning an element on a beam. First they could perform the element on the floor, then on the folded mat, and finally on the balance beam. This transition may be useful when preparing to go from a low beam to a high beam. With several transition areas, more students will be able to practice moves concurrently, eliminating or shortening lines for equipment.

MAT MAZE

This activity is a terrific one to use to encourage exploration and develop climbing skills with kindergartners and first graders. It is especially desirable for special needs children to develop these skills. To create the maze, lay two folded mats on the floor parallel to each other. Their distance apart is determined by the length of the mat that is being used. The mats that are parallel to each other should be the same length. Then on top of those two mats, lay two more mats which will be perpendicular to the original two mats. The four mats should now form a square (see figure 3.7).

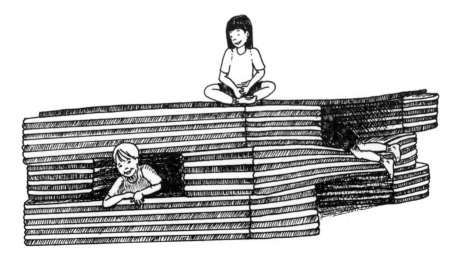

Figure 3.7   Mat Maze

Continue to stack the mats until the maze is approximately four feet tall. For larger children, the mats may need to be placed two on top of each other before changing the direction of the mats so that the hole that is formed is large enough for the children to crawl through. The bottom hole, however, could remain small because the students would be crawling along the floor to try to get through that hole. The Mat Maze can be part of an obstacle course, or it can be an area where the children remain for a predetermined length of time. It should be carefully monitored in case some of the students move the mats as they are crawling through the holes.

THE RAT RACE

The Rat Race is another type of maze formed by folded tumbling mats. Place the mats on the floor in the pattern of a maze so that there are some dead ends where the students would have to turn around to find the proper way out. There should be only one entrance and only one exit. The students enter the maze through the entrance and try to quickly get through it, exiting only through the exit (see figure 3.8). If the students trying to get through the maze run into a dead end, they must turn around and try another path to get to the exit.

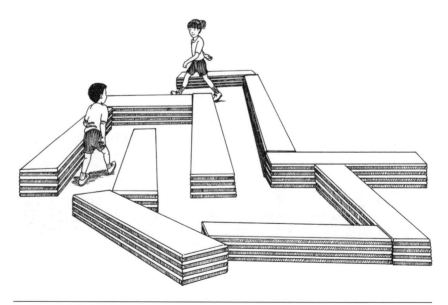

Figure 3.8   The Rat Race

Smaller students, such as pre-kindergarten and kindergarten students, should be allowed to walk through the Rat Race the first time. Taller students should crawl through the Rat Race maze to make it a little more challenging. This maze can be a station in an obstacle course, but it may need to be checked occasionally to be certain that none of the rats got frustrated and created a new exit by moving the mats.

AEROBIC STEPS

Many programs cannot afford enough aerobic steps to accommodate an entire class. Folding mats may be substituted for the aerobic steps. Several students may use a single mat, and the mats can be adjusted in height simply by unfolding one section of the folding mat to reach the desired height.

CHAPTER 4

DON'T THROW IT OUT JUST BECAUSE IT'S BROKEN!

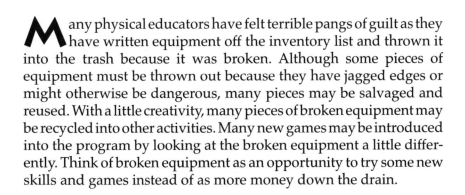

M any physical educators have felt terrible pangs of guilt as they have written equipment off the inventory list and thrown it into the trash because it was broken. Although some pieces of equipment must be thrown out because they have jagged edges or might otherwise be dangerous, many pieces may be salvaged and reused. With a little creativity, many pieces of broken equipment may be recycled into other activities. Many new games may be introduced into the program by looking at the broken equipment a little differently. Think of broken equipment as an opportunity to try some new skills and games instead of as more money down the drain.

BEADED JUMP ROPES

Occasionally beaded jump ropes do break beyond repair, or some of the beads must be removed from the rope in order to repair the jump rope. Save these plastic beads for another game called Monkey Feet. To play this game, scatter old beads from broken jump ropes all over the gym floor. The students each remove one shoe, but leave their socks on their feet. The students are not allowed to touch the beads with their hands. They must pick up the beads with their toes and drop them into the shoe that they are carrying.

The game is over when all of the beads have been picked up. A winner may be determined by counting to see who has the most beads, or the students may scatter the beads on the floor and play the game again to see whether they can pick up more beads in the second round than they picked up the first time. During the second round, the students can put on the shoe that they were carrying in the first round and take off the other shoe so that the game is a little different for them. Please note that this game will also work with packing peanuts if no jump rope beads are available.

POPPED BALLS

Many playground balls that no longer will hold air are sitting in a landfill somewhere and will be there through eternity. They were made to be durable and will not decompose, so they should be recycled once they have outlived their original purpose. One suggestion for recycling them is to cut them in half and then cut slits about every inch so that they will lay flat on the floor. You can then use them as poly spots for marking the floor.

Another suggestion is to cut the ball in half to make "it caps." Use a coffee filter inside the cap for each student, and then throw the coffee filter out to prevent any potential spread of lice. A student who is designated as "it" in a tag game may wear the "it cap" instead of a jersey. When many of these "it caps" have been accumulated, students can use them to play several games.

SHARKS AND SWIMMERS

This active tag game is designed for students who are in the fourth grade or higher. Two or three sharks are designated for the first game. All of the other students are swimmers and must wear swim caps (old playground balls that have been cut in half). Make sure each cap is lined with a coffee filter for hygiene purposes. If a swimmer is tagged by a shark, the swimmer must lay down in the place where he or she was tagged. The tagged student must then swim on his or her belly back to the shore, which is a wall assigned as the shore before the game starts. Once the shore is reached, the swimmer may return to the game.

At the end of one minute, time is called, and all swimmers must freeze wherever they are. If there are five or more swimmers down on the floor, the sharks win. If there are fewer than five swimmers on the floor, the swimmers win the round. The sharks then select someone to replace them as sharks as they then become swimmers, and the game continues until every player has had a turn to be a shark. For large classes, more sharks may be used for each game.

CONEHEADS

Use old footballs cut in half for the it caps instead of old playground balls. The players who are assigned to be "it" wear the football it caps and are called Coneheads. You should have at least two Coneheads; you may need more for a larger class. The Coneheads try to catch the other players. If someone is tagged by a Conehead, the player must hook elbows with the Conehead. When another player is tagged, that player is to hook elbows with the first player that was tagged, making a chain of players with the Conehead on the end. The game is over when all of the players have been tagged and are in the Conehead chains. The group that has the longest chain of players is the winning group. To play again, the new Coneheads would be the players who are on the end of the chains. These should be the last players who were caught. This adds some incentive to try to avoid being caught by the Coneheads.

BROKEN BADMINTON RACQUETS

Many badminton racquets have been thrown away due to broken strings. The cost of restringing the racquets is usually higher than buying another racquet; therefore, they go into the trash. A suggestion for recycling these broken racquets is to get a small, flat container and use the old racquet as a bubble wand. This activity would make a great station for a field day or just a great outside activity for spring. The racquets make a myriad of tiny bubbles that students enjoy running after and popping. Creating bubbles is even easier when there is a slight breeze outside.

SOUND PADDLES AND BEACH BALLS

If the face of a sound paddle breaks, do not throw it away. Save it until there is a beach ball that will no longer hold air. Most sound paddles are held together with screws. Take the screws out and stretch the plastic from the beach ball across the paddle. (Be sure to cut the beach ball so that there is a single layer of plastic across the paddle.) Put the paddles back together, keeping the plastic taut. Replace the screws, and you have a new functional paddle. It will no longer make the noise that it originally made, but it will be a functional paddle for a light ball such as a table tennis ball or a yarn fluff ball.

BROKEN HULA HOOPS

Broken hula hoops make excellent hurdles or obstacles for going under. Place the ends of the broken hoop into two small traffic cones, forming an arch with the hoop. The height of the hoop can be adjusted by putting the cones closer or farther apart. To incorporate these arches into an obstacle course, place several of them in a row and have the students do a crab walk or a snake crawl under them. These arches may also be substituted for hurdles when you teach a unit on track and field. In addition, they may be used for a game called Human Croquet.

To play Human Croquet, place hula hoop arches, made from broken hula hoops, in the formation of a croquet game. Place the ends of the hoops in traffic cones to form the arches, or if the game is played outside, press the ends of the hoops firmly into the ground so that they will not pop up as the children are passing under the arches. See figure 4.1. The students are timed as they perform a crawl, crab walk, bear walk, or any other locomotor skill assigned by the teacher through the course. The students may go individually or as a group, each following a leader that knows the pattern.

Another variation of this game is to have a student start at each end of the course. The students try to go through the croquet pattern and beat the other student back to his or her starting point. The game may get funny if the students happen to meet and try to get through the

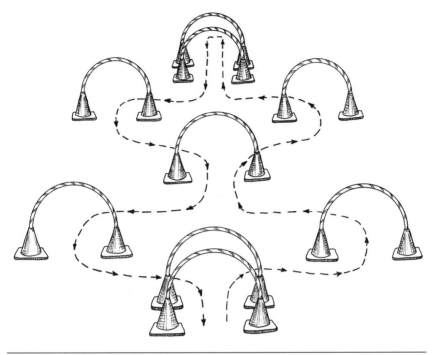

Figure 4.1 Human Croquet court

same hoop at the same time. You can also play this game with groups, but do not be surprised if some of the students in the groups get confused and end up at the wrong ending point.

OLD PINNIES OR JERSEYS

When pinnies or jerseys are getting tattered, they may be used as blindfolds in games. You can use blindfold games to develop spatial awareness, which is a necessary component of tumbling. A very simple blindfold game is for one student to try to lead a blindfolded student through an obstacle course by using verbal cues. Another use for old pinnies is to use them for flags. You can tie them to the end of a PVC pipe or broomstick and use them as marker flags for a field.

STICK-A-BALL PADDLES

For some reason, two-part stick-a-ball paddles do not like to remain together. The plastic ring always seems to separate from the paddle part. The paddle is completely functional without the ring, and it is a pesky job to keep reattaching the ring to the paddle. Keep those rings to use for a ring toss game. Set up several cones for the students to try to throw the rings onto. Set a hula hoop on the ground so that the students know where to stand when throwing the rings. Several hoops may be set up so that several students may be tossing rings at the same time. It may be helpful to color-coordinate the rings with the hula hoops. The students will have fewer conflicts over the rings if the blue ring goes to the blue hoop, and the yellow ring goes to the yellow hoop, and so on.

FLAT TENNIS BALLS

Flat tennis balls are useful when practicing throwing accuracy, whether overhand or underhand. They make excellent objects for throwing at targets, but they are especially effective in a game called Bonus Ball. This game is designed for older elementary students, such as fourth, fifth, or sixth graders who are beginning to play team-oriented games. The students are divided into teams of two, three, or four players. Each of the teams is assigned a different number. In a box, the teacher has five tennis balls for each team that are marked with the team's number. There are also several bonus balls in the box. The bonus balls may be marked with a star, or they may have no markings on them at all, which would distinguish them from the other balls as well.

The teacher dumps the box so that all of the balls scatter throughout the gym. When the teacher calls for the children to start, the first team member from each team must run out and find a ball with the team's number on it. When the student finds a correct ball, the student returns to the group with the ball. Then the next student may go look for one of the team's balls. After the team has located and returned all five of its numbered balls, the players may begin to look for and return bonus balls. A student is only allowed to bring back one ball from the floor on each turn.

The team that retrieves the most balls is the winning team. All of the balls are then returned to the box, and the teacher can scatter them again to start another game. A variation of the game is to have each team find five balls in numerical order. The first player would have to return with a ball that is marked 1, the second player would have to return with a ball marked 2, and so on until the team had all five balls. The players would then be allowed to search for the bonus balls.

OLD RACQUETBALLS

Old racquetballs never die, they just get a slit in them or lose their bounce. Either way, they make perfect clown noses. With a small slit in them, they can stick on the end of most noses. Just squeeze the ball so the slit opens wide, and then close it on the end of a nose. This prop is great for playing Clown Tag. The people who are designated as the clowns wear a racquetball on the end of their noses. When a clown tags another student, the student must perform the circus stunt that is selected prior to the round of tag before the student may reenter the game. This game should be a two-ring circus: the clown and the students trying not to get tagged should be on one side of the floor (one ring), and the stunt performers should be on the other side of the floor (the other ring).

Try these suggested circus stunts:

1. Do five log rolls. (Be sure to have a folding mat out in the ring for this stunt.)
2. Do two forward rolls. (Be sure to have a folding mat out for this stunt.)
3. Do 20 steps in an elephant walk.
4. Do 20 steps in a bear walk.
5. Do the split (the best one possible) and count to 10.
6. Put both hands on the floor and kick both feet up together in a donkey kick.
7. Do the seal walk across the floor.
8. Do 10 jumps with a jump rope on one foot.
9. Stand on one foot while counting to 10.
10. Take 20 steps on tiptoes.

OLD MISCELLANEOUS EQUIPMENT AND BALLS

Many schools require the physical education teacher to select students to receive awards at the conclusion of the school year. Any old, no longer useful equipment could be used for making awards. Smaller equipment such as golf balls, table tennis paddles, tennis balls, gloves, or pieces of a larger piece of equipment, such as a net, would make great awards for the end of the year. Here are some suggested awards you could hand out:

1. Good Sportsmanship Award
2. Tenacity Award
3. Most Improved Overall
4. Most Improved in . . . . .
5. Most Helpful to Others Award
6. Physical Fitness Award

To make the awards, paint the piece of equipment that is being used for the award with silver or gold spray paint. Mount the piece to a board with a glue gun so that it will sit on a shelf. If the item is free-standing, a board may not be necessary. Either way, after the paint has dried, add an inscription by using fabric paints or by using a file label. Type the inscription on the label, and then peel and stick the label on the board or equipment piece. The students will treasure these handmade awards.

CHAPTER 5

ACQUIRING FREE EQUIPMENT

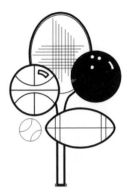

Free equipment is available to schools; however, acquiring free equipment is an art. There are many methods of acquiring equipment: some equipment is just there waiting to be taken, and other equipment requires a little more effort to obtain. Some equipment acquisitions require having the parents collect UPCs or proofs of purchase, but most require no money for shipping and handling charges. This chapter is divided into three sections: equipment that is absolutely free, equipment you can acquire with proofs of purchase, and general budget stretching ideas.

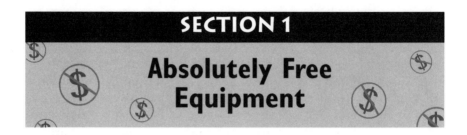

SECTION 1

Absolutely Free Equipment

Acquiring free equipment is often an exciting process. Many sources are available for free equipment and these that are mentioned are certainly not the only ones available. Hopefully, they will serve as a springboard for other ideas of sources that may be available within individual communities. The ideas that follow will be a great starting point for finding free equipment.

CARPET SQUARES

Carpet squares are magnificent additions to an equipment supply. They are versatile; you can use them for anything from marking personal spaces to playing games. Most carpet dealers have plenty of these squares, but they would prefer to sell them for around a dollar each. Many people come begging for them, from day care providers to churches. Getting these squares for free requires an unusual approach and a sense of humor. "The Pancake Theory" is one approach that usually works.

Explain to the owner or manager which school needs the squares for their physical education program. Tell him it has something to do with "The Pancake Theory." The theory is that kindergarten children seem to possess a magnetic property that draws them together until they are stacked like pancakes. These carpet squares, however, seem to somehow demagnetize them, allowing them to stay in one place where they may participate in physical education without being stacked together. Usually the owner or manager will enjoy your unique approach and sense of humor and ask how many you would like. Do not be greedy! Do not try to get an entire class set from one dealer. Ask if 10 or 12 would be acceptable. The owner may offer more than that; certainly take anything that is offered. If you aren't greedy, the dealer may be willing to help again when you need more squares later on.

Carpet squares have a variety of functions. You can use them to mark spaces for children. When the children play tag games where they need to scatter and then return to a safe area, the squares can be the safe areas. You also can use the squares to introduce step aerobics. Instead of using a step, each student has a carpet square. The children can then concentrate on how to use the step and follow the instructor without the extra work of learning to use a real step. After they seem to be able to follow a step aerobic session with the carpet squares, a real step may be introduced.

You also may use carpet squares for games and activities that will be popular with students. These carpet square games and activities may include the following:

1. Students can put a carpet square under each foot and skate across the floor and back to the starting place.

2. Each player has two squares. The player must stand on one square and toss the other square. The player then steps onto the empty square, picks up the first square, and tosses it. When the player reaches the other side of the room, he or she may pick up the squares and run back to the starting point.

3. One square is used for three players in a group. One player sits on the square while two other players hold on to one of the sitting player's hands. They pull the sitting player to the other side of the room and back. Each member of the group should receive a turn as the rider on the square.

4. With both hands remaining on the carpet square, the player pushes it to the other side of the room and back.

5. Each player receives a plunger and a carpet square. The player must kneel on the square and reach ahead with the plunger, sticking it on the floor. The player moves ahead by pulling on the stick of the plunger, pulling the plunger off the floor, and reattaching it farther up the floor. When the player gets to the other side, he or she may pick up the square and run back to the starting point.

6. With one foot on a carpet square and the other foot on the floor, the student steps and slides across the room and back.

7. With both feet on the carpet square, the student twists and scoots across the floor while standing. Upon reaching the other side, the student may run back to the starting point.

8. Each student is given four carpet squares. The student must keep a hand or a foot on each of the four squares to slide across the room and back.

STUFFED ANIMALS

Stuffed animals are easily accumulated by sending a note home to the parents stating that you need old stuffed animals that they no longer want. Explain that you will be using them to expand the physical education program. You can use stuffed animals to expand the possibilities for hand-eye coordination activities, foot-eye coordination activities, and obstacle courses. Stuffed animals also make wonderful targets when practicing throwing techniques.

ANIMAL OBSTACLE COURSE

Most kindergarten classes study animals during the school year. Adding an animal obstacle course at that time truly enhances the unit. First and second graders will also enjoy the course. This activity is a delightful way to practice basic locomotor skills for these younger children. To set up an exciting course, all you need are some stuffed animals and some white contact paper.

The course is determined by the animals that are acquired. The animals are spread over the length of the floor where the children are to do a particular motor activity. For instance, if the children are supposed to do the elephant walk for 12 feet, and there are three stuffed elephants, place an animal at the 1-foot, 6-foot, and 12-foot marks. Cut appropriate animal footprints out of the contact paper and stick them to the floor. The children follow the elephant prints for the 12 feet, as well as following the other visual cues of the stuffed animals. With the animals and the footprints, the children rarely get confused about what to do or how far to do it.

The following list explains how you can use some animals that are commonly donated:

- *Bears.* The children should walk on hands and feet, keeping the legs straight. Make bear claws from the contact paper.
- *Rabbits.* Most likely many rabbits will appear from past Easter celebrations. You can use them to make an area for two-foot jumping.

- *Monkeys.* Monkeys scratch and roll and act silly. Most children will easily adapt to this area.
- *Birds.* If a balance beam is available, have the children walk across the beam. The beam can simulate a fence that a bird might rest upon or a telephone wire where birds like to gather.
- *Cats and Dogs.* The children may crawl through this area, selecting which animal they would rather imitate. They should make the noise of that animal while going through the area.

With any luck, some other, more unusual animals will be donated. Some of those animals may include the following:

- *Spiders.* The children perform a crab walk through this area.
- *Snakes.* Children slither on the floor through the snake pit area.
- *Frogs.* Children squat low to perform a frog leap, landing in a squat.
- *Storks.* The children balance on one foot for as long as possible. When the other foot touches the floor, the children move on to the next area.
- *Seals.* The children pull themselves along with their arms, dragging their straight legs behind them.
- *Kangaroos.* Children do two-foot jumping for distance in this area.
- *Horses.* Children gallop in this area.
- *Elephants.* The children clasp their hands together to form a trunk from their arms. They bend over forward swinging their hands near to the floor. This position is supposed to resemble an elephant searching the floor for peanuts.
- *Dinosaurs, sharks, and other odd animals.* Establish a petting zoo or aquariam for animals that either do not have any other like them or that are too strange to adapt to an area; if you want, you can create a fenced area for the petting zoo from folded mats; an old wading pool is ideal for creating an aquarium. In this area, the children may pet any of the animals, including those in the aquarium. Children need to touch things, and this area allows a place for them to touch and feel the stuffed animals. The children are unlikely to

touch any of the animals that are set up to identify a skill area in the obstacle course, so the petting zoo area is important. It also provides a place in the obstacle course for oversized or unusual animals that have been donated. This place may be important to the child who donated an odd animal.

BALLOONS

Balloons are easy to find. They are located at grand openings, reopening celebrations, sales, parades, car lots, festivals, and just about anywhere that there is a special event or a crowd. Banks and restaurants give them away to children. Most people working at these functions would prefer to give someone a handful of balloons to be inflated and used later in a physical education program, rather than inflate them themselves. Consider that these people have probably been inflating balloons for hours, and as soon as the balloons are gone, they may get to stop. Such a person will be most pleasant about handing out a few balloons that are not inflated. Save these balloons until there are enough to use for games or relays. You could probably find enough balloons throughout the school year to use for balloon popping races at a field day event.

BOWLING PINS

Most bowling alleys throw out old bowling pins. They would be delighted to donate them to a school to use for physical education classes. Not only could these pins be used to introduce the students to bowling, they may be useful in other games such as Kick-Pin Ball. This game is similar to baseball and should be played by the older students, fourth grade or higher, who are beginning to work on team games.

Divide the class into two teams. One is the kicking team, and the other is the fielding team. The field is set up similar to baseball, except the bases are closer together. The bases should be approximately 15 to 20 feet apart. A playground ball is used for the game. Each of the bases, including the home plate, has a bowling pin set slightly in front of the base. The fielding team places a player at each of the bases. These base players stand over the bowling pin in a straddled position.

The pitcher, who is on the fielding team, rolls the ball to the kicker. The kicker should kick the ball as far as possible; no bunting is allowed in this game. The kicker then runs behind the bases in a counter-clockwise direction. The kicker does not have to touch any of the bases, merely run behind each of the bases and return to touch the home plate. The fielding team must recover the kicked ball (the pitcher is not allowed to be the first to recover a kicked ball) and throw it to the player on first base. The first base player knocks down the bowling pin between his or her legs with the ball. The first base player then proceeds to throw the ball to the second base player, who knocks over the bowling pin in the same manner. The ball is then thrown to the third base player who likewise knocks over the bowling pin located there. Finally, the ball is thrown to the player at the home plate, who knocks over the bowling pin that is there.

The kicking team scores a run if the kicker makes it back to the home plate before the bowling pin at the home plate is knocked over. If the fielding teams gets all of the pins knocked over before the runner makes it back to the home plate, an out occurs. The fielding team may not get a runner out by hitting him or her with the ball. An out only occurs by knocking the pins over faster than the kicker runs around the bases. After three outs occur, the teams switch places. The kicking order remains the same so that all players get a turn to kick the ball during the game.

The students should be instructed to simply knock the pin down so that it merely falls over when they play a base. They should not attempt to hit the pin with the ball so that the pin shoots across the floor. A flying pin could possibly hit or trip a runner. The base players should simply bend forward and tap the top of the bowling pin with the ball and throw the ball on to the next base player. If the students follow these guidelines, the pin merely tips over with no danger to the runner.

GOLF TUBES

Golf tubes are the long, plastic tubes that protect golf clubs when they are being shipped. Any store that sells golf clubs, usually a golf specialty shop or a pro shop at a golf course, will have more of these tubes than they know what to do with. They must discard them in order to display sets of clubs to sell. These tubes are quite sturdy and flexible and make excellent additions to the physical education supply room.

You can use these tubes as substitutes for more expensive tinikling sticks. Because these tubes are hollow, you can use them as a percussion instrument when performing rhythmic activities. Students can hold the tubes as a balance wand as they walk across a low balance beam, imitating a tightrope walker from the circus. Golf tubes also make superb boundary markers when you lay them end-to-end on the floor or the ground. In addition, they make excellent flagpoles. Because they are lightweight, they would be ideal flagpoles for students to carry in a march for a field day parade. If each class makes a flag to represent their class, they could mount the flag on one of these golf tubes and have the leaders carry the flags. Golf tubes are also perfect for practicing balancing and throwing skills and playing games.

HORIZONTAL BALANCING SKILLS

Holding the tube in a horizontal position, students attempt to balance the tube in the following ways:

1. On the back of the hand
2. On the palm of the hand
3. On the forehead
4. On top of the head
5. On the nose
6. On one shoulder
7. On the forearm
8. On a foot that is held in the air
9. On a knee that is held in the air
10. On the back while bending forward

VERTICAL BALANCING SKILLS

Holding the tube in a vertical position, students attempt to repeat the 10 horizontal balancing skills. Add locomotor skills to the balancing skills if the students have mastered some of the balancing skills. The students could walk 10 steps forward or backward while balancing the tube on the back of the hand. Combining locomotor skills and the plastic tubes leads to endless possibilities for challenges.

STACKING TUBES

The ends of the tubes may be compressed so that they fit into the end of another tube. Place the students in groups of three or four to see how many tubes they can stack in this fashion to build a tower. If the tower falls, they may start over. Give a time period for this activity, and at the conclusion of the time period, approximately five to ten minutes, let them observe the stacks created by the other groups. The tubes are flexible and durable and will withstand the bending that this activity requires. They will quickly spring back into their original shapes.

JAVELIN THROW

The tubes may be used to practice techniques for the javelin throw. To prevent problems in retrieving the tubes, number the tubes with permanent marker. This numbering eliminates arguments about whose tube is whose. Also, be sure to have all students throwing and then retrieving the tubes at the same time. For safety purposes, no students should be retrieving tubes while others are throwing them. During the fall when the children are studying Native Americans, this activity is an excellent one to do because Native Americans used to have spear throwing contests. Contests were held for distance and for accuracy. To throw the tubes for accuracy, place several batting T's or other objects for targets in the gym or the field and let the students venture to hit the targets with the tubes as they pretend to hunt for food such as rabbits and birds.

TOILET PAPER

Being friendly to the janitors certainly has benefits, for rolls of toilet paper can come in handy as equipment in the gym. The janitors are usually willing to spare some rolls when they see the fun and frolic that is dispatched with them. Rolls of toilet paper that are still in their original condition make a funny substitute for traffic cones when constructing hurdles from broken hula hoops. Stack two rolls of toilet paper on top of each other and insert one end of the broken hula hoop into the toilet paper. Then do the same on the other side. These hurdles are sure to bring a chuckle to the students. Rolls of toilet paper are also the primary piece of equipment for a game called Wrap the Mummy.

This game is perfect for playing during the week of Halloween. It emphasizes teamwork and cooperative effort and is best for students who are in the fourth grade or higher. This game lasts approximately 10 minutes. To get the game going, divide the students into groups of three and give each group a roll of toilet paper. The group must select one of the members to be the mummy. Each group tries to wrap their mummy so that it is the best-looking mummy; the paper should cover all of the person's parts. No tape is allowed, and the students must configure a method of concealing the end of the paper.

Inform the students that it is acceptable to leave a breathing hole for the mummy. Also inform them that once the mummy can no longer see, it will be difficult for the person playing the part of the mummy to keep his or her balance. They will then be responsible for keeping the mummy from falling and tearing the paper. Also encourage the students to add creative touches, such as sunglasses or jewelry to the mummies. Emphasize that time is not a major factor; the groups should work for quality rather than speed. There are no bonus points given for being the first group to finish.

The contest may end by one of two methods. Each group may continue until they have completely used up the roll of toilet paper that they were given, or the groups must all stop at the end of a given time period, approximately seven minutes. At that time, someone who is impartial should judge the mummies to see which one is the best-looking mummy. If the classroom teacher is able to return a couple of minutes early, he or she will get a great laugh from this activity and would be a great judge. If the teacher is unable to return to be the judge, a janitor, cafeteria worker, office staff member, or someone who happens to be in the halls would be acceptable for a judge. After the best mummy has been decided, the groups must tear away the paper from the mummy. (See some of the clean-up games suggested in the "Old Newspapers" section of chapter 2.)

JAR OPENERS

Jar openers are those rubber gripping items that are usually round and are designed to assist people in opening those difficult-to-open jars. They often contain the logo of a company that is somehow related to homes, such as a real estate company or a home repair company. They are frequently given out at home and patio shows and can sometimes be found at street festivals. Most companies will be willing to donate several of them if they realize that the openers are going to be used to play games in a physical education class. These jar openers are terrific substitutes for the more expensive items known as poly spots.

Jar openers often come in a variety of colors so that games requiring different groups can be color-coded. Groups of children may be color-coded to match the jar openers so that they can be told to go to the jar opener that corresponds to their color. If the jar openers are identical, you can differentiate them by coloring them with a permanent marker. You can turn white jar openers into any color you want. If the colors of the jar openers are too dark to change, you could add polka dots or stripes to them.

You could also cut the openers to form a variety of shapes to distinguish the groups. The various colors or shapes could also stand for different activities to be performed. For example, you could cut them to make footprints for the animal obstacle course that can be stored and used from year to year instead of the disposable ones made from contact paper.

PLASTIC BUCKETS

You can find five-gallon plastic buckets throughout the community. Items that are sold in bulk, such as laundry detergent and pickles, are often packaged in these large plastic buckets. These buckets can be useful in many areas, ranging from storing small pieces of equipment to being the sole pieces of equipment required for games. Because these buckets have handles, they work wonderfully for transporting small pieces of equipment such as tennis balls. The buckets also are great for storing equipment that does not stack very well.

Be sure to thoroughly wash, rinse, and dry the buckets prior to using them for game equipment. Do not stack the buckets together until they are absolutely dry. If they are stacked together while they are still damp, a vacuum may be created that will make it very difficult to separate the buckets later. Also note that some of the buckets may have holes in the bottom. Use these buckets to store equipment or for a game known as Bucket Feet. For games that require water, make sure you use the buckets that do not have holes in them.

BUCKET FEET

This game develops balance and coordination; it is also a good field day activity. Each player is given two buckets. The players hold the handles of the buckets with their hands. With their feet in the buckets, the players walk or run to the turning point and back to the starting point. A variation of this game requires only one bucket. The players stand with both feet in the bucket and hold the handle in front of the legs. The players then jump inside the bucket to the turning point and back. Students could also learn a simple line dance to be performed with their feet in buckets. This performance would require concentration, coordination, and balance.

BOBBING FOR APPLES

This excellent field day activity provides an opportunity for the children to cool off and to have a refreshing snack during the activities. If a local grocer is not willing to donate the apples for this special day, parents who would like to volunteer time but are unable to due to other responsibilities are often willing to send in a bag or two of apples. Many parents would like to contribute to these activities and would appreciate having a chance to help in some way, even though they cannot physically be there.

Bobbing for Apples is done a little differently than the traditional dumping of all of the apples into one bucket. In order to prevent children from trying to bite into an apple that several other children have already tried to bite, the participant picks the apple and drops it in the bucket, which is approximately two-thirds full of water. After four or five dunks into the water attempting to pick up the apple with the teeth, the participant may reach into the water and take the apple out with the hands. The children will be delighted with this activity, yet surprised at how difficult it is to retrieve the apple with only the teeth. Set up several buckets for apple bobbing so that the children will not have to wait in lines to participate.

SPONGE RACE

The Sponge Race is definitely an outdoor activity and is a most appropriate field day activity. This race is for teams of three or four people. A bucket filled with water is approximately 15 feet away from every team. The team stands in a line facing the bucket of water. At the starting signal, the first person in the line runs to the bucket and saturates the sponge in the water. The player runs back to the front of the line and the players must pass the sponge overhead until it reaches the last person in the line. The last person then takes the sponge to the water bucket and drenches it. The player then goes to the front of the line and passes it until it reaches the last person again. This process continues until everyone in the line has had a chance to take the sponge to the water bucket or until everyone is thoroughly soaked!

TWO BUCKET RACE

This outdoor relay game is another excellent activity for field day. Any number of teams may play at the same time, but at least two teams are needed. Teams should consist of two or three players so that each person is constantly in motion. Each team has a bucket full of water at the front of the line. The teams also have a bucket at the end of the line that is empty. The first player in the line has a cup and upon hearing the starting signal, fills the cup and passes it down the line. The last player dumps the water into the empty bucket and runs to the front of the line to fill the cup and begin the passing process again. At the end of a given time period (approximately five minutes will be enough to thoroughly soak all of the players), the team that has the most water in the bucket at the end of the line wins the game.

WATER SHUTTLE RACE

Each player in this game is given a large cup and a small cup. The large cup is placed on the ground at the starting point, which is approximately 10 feet away from the water bucket. The players carry the small cup to the bucket of water and fill the small cup. They quickly return to the large cup and dump the water into it. The players continue to run back and forth between the water bucket and their large cups until one of the players has completely filled the large cup. The first player to fill the large cup wins the game.

CHICKEN SOUP

You can change the name of this game to Rabbit Stew, Duck Soup, Bear Stew, or any other name according to what stuffed animals or objects are available for playing. For Chicken Soup, divide the students into groups of three or four. Each group has three or four rubber chickens or stuffed animal chickens and an empty plastic bucket. The bucket is the soup kettle and is placed approximately 15 to 20 feet from the players. The students throw the chickens at the kettle. Each time an animal makes it into the kettle, the entire group scores a point. After all of the animals have been thrown, the students retrieve them and throw again. The students continue to play and add to their score until the teacher calls for the end of the throwing. A winner may be determined by which group got the most meat into the soup. This game is funnier if stuffed vegetables are also available to throw at the kettle. However, real vegetables are not recommended for this game.

PAPER PLATES

Paper plates are wonderful pieces of equipment for physical education programs. In fact, you can hold an event called the Paper Plate Olympics and fill an entire day with activities that require paper plates. You may be able to acquire paper plates left over from a school function or convince a local restaurant to donate some. Otherwise, you can purchase them very inexpensively from a discount store. The cheapest, thinnest plates are acceptable for these games.

PAPER PLATE OLYMPICS

Although many games are listed under this topic, some are more appropriate for younger children, and some should be used only with older children. Most of the activities, however, are exciting for children of all ages.

1. **Discus Throw**. The students throw the paper plate using the style of throwing a discus or the style of throwing a Frisbee. The students attempt to get the discus as far as possible down the field or the gym. Give the students several chances to practice this skill before competing.

2. **Cross-Country Run.** The students cross their legs and keep them crossed throughout the entire race. They hold the paper plate either on top of their heads or behind their backs with both hands as they run to the turning point and then back to the starting point. This awkward race is fun to participate in and fun to watch.

3. **The Back Stroke.** The students hold the paper plate behind their backs as they run to the turning point and return to the starting line. To hold the plates on their backs, the students must put one hand over the head and then reach to the center of the back. The other hand goes behind the back and reaches upward to join the paper plate. The students must run the entire distance holding the plate this way.

4. **Mixed Pairs.** In this game, students must find someone to be their partners by running and joining elbows with another person and holding the paper plates against their stomachs with the hand of the free arm. (This hand may change as the game progresses and pairs are switched.) If another player joins arms with one of the members of the pair, the other member must let go and run to join another pair. The pairs are free to move around the room. When the teacher calls out for the students to stop, all of the students must stay where they are. Any students who are not joined to another person, or any students that have three joined together at that moment, must perform a stunt. Some suggested stunts include the following:

   a. Whistle the alphabet song.
   b. Sing the Happy Birthday song to the teacher.
   c. Leapfrog over everyone else.
   d. Pretend to be a hippopotamus performing a ballet dance.
   e. Lean forward, putting both hands on the floor, and kick their feet up together three times while saying, "Hee haw."
   f. Spin around eight times and then run across the room.
   g. Do the Russian dance.
   h. Do a hula dance.

5. **Bobsled Race.** Each bobsled team consists of three members. With all players standing and facing the same direction, the first holds a paper plate in front like a steering wheel. The second player holds a paper plate against the back of the first player. The third player holds a paper plate against the back of the second player. Members of the bobsled team must not become disconnected from the player(s) in front of them. When the first player reaches

the turning point, all three of the players turn around to face the starting point. The first player is now the last member, the middle member remains the middle member, and the last player is now the driver with the steering plate. The team returns to the starting point in this new order.

6. **High Jump.** Each player holds his or her paper plate in front of him or her with the right hand on the right side of the plate and the left hand on the left side. The players lean forward and attempt to jump with both feet simultaneously over the paper plate without letting go of the paper plate. Younger children may need to jump over with one foot at a time. Letting go of the plate is acceptable if the student loses his or her balance while performing this activity.

7. **Raceway.** Each student holds the paper plate as a steering wheel and runs about the room without crashing into another car. If the students do crash into another car, both students involved in the crash must lay down on their backs, tuck their knees to their chest, and rock back and forth as they count to 10. This rocking represents being repaired at the body shop. After counting to 10 in this position, the students may return to the game. After one crash, the students who have been to the repair shop must hop on one foot as they drive through the room. If they have a second crash after going to the repair shop, the car must then move about the room on the knees only. If a car crashes for a third time, the car is towed by the teacher to the scrap yard where the car may remain until the end of the game (or until the teacher returns them as recycled scrap metal). This punishment discourages students from deliberately running into other students.

8. **Long Jump.** The students squat down and hold the paper plate in front of the shins. Holding the plate in this way should help the students keep their bottoms down while jumping. They jump three times to see how far they can go on three jumps without standing between the jumps. The winner is the student who can travel the farthest on three jumps.

9. **Skating.** Each student is given two paper plates and places them on the floor. With one foot on each of the paper plates,

the students skate through the room. You can hold races, or the children may have fun just skating around the room.

10. **Inchworm Races.** Each student is given two paper plates. One is placed on the floor slightly in front of the students. The student leans forward, placing both hands on the paper plate. The other paper plate is placed under both feet. The students make forward progress by pushing the hands forward and then pulling the feet forward, keeping both the hands and the feet on their plates. The students resemble inchworms as they progress across the floor. You may do this activity as a race or as a relay.

11. **Crab Races.** The students must balance their paper plates on their stomachs as they do the crab walk for this race. This race may be performed as a relay activity. To add a little variety to the race, have the students do the crab walk forward to the turning point and then do the crab walk backward to the starting point.

12. **Waiter Races.** In this race, the students balance two paper plates, one with each hand, as they proceed to the finish line as quickly as they can. If a paper plate falls, it must be returned to the student's hands before that student may proceed.

13. **Duck Races.** The students hold the paper plate against their bottoms or their shins as they perform the duck walk for the duration of the race.

14. **Equestrian Races.** The students hold the paper plates as reins as they gallop for the duration of the race.

15. **Breast Stroke.** The students hold the paper plate against their chests with their chins as they race to the turning point and back. The plate may not be held with the hands. If it is dropped, the student must stop to return the plate to his or her chest using his or her hands before proceeding.

These examples are just some of the many possible activities for the Paper Plate Olympics, which would be most appropriate during an Olympic year when the students are getting excited about the worldwide games. This event would introduce the younger children to the nature of an Olympic festival where a variety of games are played.

HIDE AND SEEK

This game is fun to play around Easter when the children are excited about hunting and seeking games. Each group should consist of two or three players so that the players have a moment to catch their breath before running again. This game is best for students who are in the third grade or older and are beginning to participate in some team-oriented games. For each group, there should be six paper plates. Each group is assigned a color, and the six paper plates that belong to that group will have a circle of that color in the center of the paper plate. There should also be six blank paper plates just for fun. The paper plates are scattered all over the floor and are mixed up and upside down so that no one may see what color circle is on the plate.

Upon the starting signal, one student from each group runs out onto the floor and turns over a paper plate. If the color on the plate corresponds to the group's color, the student takes the plate back to the group, and the next student runs out onto the floor and peeks at a paper plate. If the color does not match the group's color, the student replaces it on the floor with the color unseen. If a student draws a paper plate that has no color, he or she will also leave it on the floor upside down so that the others will not know that it is one of the blank plates. The first group to find and retrieve all six of its plates is the winner of the game.

FEED BAGS

Burlap sacks are difficult to find, but old feed sacks that are made from a heavy paper are relatively easy to locate. Most any stable or kennel should be able to supply these bags. When the bags do wear out, they are recyclable; they are considered the same as cardboard or paper bag material in most areas. Feed bags are useful for transporting equipment when it is necessary to carry several items, such as bats and ball. They also make great storage bags for larger items.

OLD TIRES

Not only are most tire companies more than willing to give tires to a school, they are often willing to deliver them as well. Often these companies are required to pay a disposal fee for placing tires in a landfill or dump because they do not deteriorate. Many companies would prefer to deliver them to a school for free rather than have to pay to deliver them to another disposal site. Be sure to ask for tires that are not steel-belted; steel-belted tires may have steel splinters sticking out of them that could injure a child. When the tires arrive, be sure to examine them to be certain that none of them is steel-belted or has any rough edges. The tires may be dirty when they arrive and may need to be cleaned before using them in any games or activities where the tires may come in contact with the children.

Old tires are very versatile. You can place them in a field to mark a running track. The students run to the outside of the tires. You can cut the old tires in half and use them for hurdles, as in figure 5.1. This activity is recommended for children in the fourth grade or higher; younger children should not participate in this activity because they are too small for jumping over the hurdles. Place several half-tires in a row and have the children run and jump over each one. To add some excitement to the activities, paint or decorate the tires.

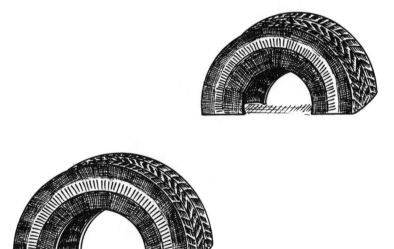

Figure 5.1 Tire hurdles

TIRE ROLL

The students can roll the tires to develop upper body strength. Be sure to use smaller tires for the younger children. They can roll them as a race or relay, or they can roll them through some sort of obstacle course. They could weave the tires around cones or other tires that are placed on the ground.

JUMPING

Old tires are also fun to jump on. One or two students at a time can stand on the tires and jump to develop leg strength. Put together several tires and place an old mattress over the tires to make a great jumping area. The students could start on one end of the mattress and jump to the other end where they would jump off.

BOOT CAMP DRILL

Place the tires in two rows end-to-end. See figure 5.2. The students have to run through the rows of tires placing one foot in every tire. Use this activity in an obstacle course or as part of field day.

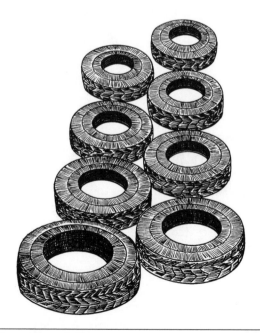

Figure 5.2 Boot camp drill

JELLY BELLY RUN

This activity is recommended for children who are in the fourth grade or higher, who are able to carry the tires in this fashion. Each student steps inside a tire and picks it up holding it so that it stays around his or her waist. The student must run to the finish line carrying the tire around the stomach.

VOLLEYBALL NET STANDARDS

These require a little work, but are well worth the effort if your program cannot afford net standards. Each standard requires an old tire, some cardboard, a flange union (you can find this at a plumbing supply store; make sure you purchase a galvanized one to prevent rust), a four-foot length of pressure-treated 2 x 4 lumber, an eight-foot length of OD pipe (this also may be found at a plumbing supply store), and two to three bags of ready-mix concrete. First, cut a circle of cardboard to fit inside the bottom of the tire. Then, cut the wood to fit inside the tire forming an X. Nail through the tire into the wood to secure the lumber. Then nail the wood together at the intersection. Screw a two-inch flange union to the intersection of the wood to accommodate a two-inch pipe standard. After placing the pipe inside the flange, mix the concrete and pour it into the tire. Allow the concrete to set for 24 hours before attempting to move the standard. You may drill holes into the pipe to attach the net to the pipe. If preferred, substitute pressure-treated lumber for the pipe and nails for the flanges. You can then use eye screws to attach the net to the standard.

OLD BROOMS

Old brooms are useful items to have in the equipment closet. You can use them for limbo sticks or tinikling sticks. The handles may be cut to make wands, lummi sticks, batons, bats, jump rope handles, line markers, or flagpoles.

BROOM GAMES AND ACTIVITIES

These activities are appropriate to implement around Halloween. Just the appearance of the old brooms will be exciting for the children. Some suggested activities include the following:

1. **Broom Ride.** The students ride the brooms to the turning point and back as if the brooms were hobby horses.

2. **Falling off the Broom.** The students hold the brooms overhead as they run pretending that they were riding the brooms and have fallen off. They hold onto the broom for dear life.

3. **Broom Bus.** Every student in the group, no more than three students to a group, straddles the broom and rides to the turning point and back to the starting point.

4. **Pumpkin Sweep.** The students sweep a basketball around the turning point and back to the beginning.

5. **Sweep the Gourd.** Instead of using a basketball, the students sweep a football to the turning point and back to the beginning.

6. **Poke the Pumpkin.** One student rolls a basketball to another student. The student with the broom attempts to stop the basketball with the broom.

7. **Scarecrow Run.** Holding the broom across the back of the shoulders with both arms straight out along the broomstick, the students must run to the turning point and back. They should look like scarecrows as they run.

8. **Shoot the Moon.** Each team is given a Frisbee that is supposed to be a full moon. The players push the Frisbee, which is upside-down on the floor, with the stick end of the broom to the turning point and back.

BROOM HOCKEY

If you have enough brooms for each of the students to have one, the class may play broom hockey. Instead of a hockey puck, a plastic beach ball is used to play this game. Divide the class into two teams with one player on each end of the gym who is the goalie. If the class is large, two people may play the goalie position for each team. Mark the goal with two cones. If the ball passes between the two cones, a point is scored for the opposite team. The wall is considered to be a neutral player. If the ball hits the wall or the bleachers and bounces off, it is still in play, just as if it had been hit by another player. No player may hit the ball above the waist. In addition to these rules, you should follow the rules of ice hockey or field hockey.

BROOM BALL

This game is played with teams. If the class is small, you can divide it into four teams and place each team in a different corner of the gym. Each team is given a broom and a milk crate. The milk crate is turned on its side so that the opening faces the center of the gym. In the center of the gym are 32 tennis balls. Eight of them are marked with the number one, eight with two, eight with three, and eight with four. Each corner of the gym also has a number. The team that is in corner number one must retrieve all eight balls that say number one and sweep them into their milk crate without ever touching the tennis balls with the hands. The players go one at a time, passing the broom to the next player when the first player has successfully swept the tennis ball into the crate. The players may only retrieve one tennis ball at a time. The first team to get all eight balls into the crate wins the game. If a ball rolls out of the crate, only the player who possesses the broom can return it to the crate.

THE WRIST TWIST

The wrist twist is a device made from a broomstick, some string, and a large fishing weight. The string is tied to the center of the broomstick and attached to the weight. The students hold their arms straight ahead of their bodies. Keeping the arms straight, the students use their wrists to turn the broomstick until the weight reaches the broomstick. This event may be timed from when the weight leaves the floor, touches the broomstick, or returns again to the floor. If several of these devices are available, the students may challenge each other to see who can go the fastest.

PLASTIC DRINKING STRAWS

Plastic drinking straws are a very inexpensive item that may be donated by a local restaurant. Look for a restaurant that does not have them wrapped individually before asking them to donate them. First of all, they will be less expensive for the merchant who is donating them if they are not individually wrapped, and secondly, they will be immediately useful with no extra work.

Straws may be used as mile markers when students are walking or jogging. Every time they pass the starting point they are given a straw. This is an easy method of tabulating the number of laps each student has completed. If a class is calculating the number of miles they accumulate in a given period, the straws could be very helpful. At the end of the jogging period, the class would put all of their straws in a marked box. The teacher could then calculate the total number of laps that were accumulated that day and translate that into the total number of miles gained by the class.

Straws also make excellent imitation javelins or spears for throwing. The students throw the straws to see who can make them go the farthest. All students must throw their straws before they all go to retrieve them so that no students would be hit by a straw. A winner will be difficult to determine because none of the straws will go very far, yet the students will enjoy trying.

OLD BICYCLE TIRES

Old bicycle tires are like old car tires. Most bicycle shops will gladly donate them. They may not deliver them to the school, but they will be glad to furnish any old tires that they may have. The tires may be used for playing two-person tug-of-war. The tug-of-war may be done with the hands pulling the tire or with the feet inside the tire to do the pulling. Bicycle tires may be hung to be used as targets for students to attempt to toss items such as bean bags or Frisbees through. The tires themselves may be thrown as giant rings to ring traffic cones with, or the students may throw the tires at a partner to attempt to ring the partner. Students may also use the tires as a Pogo stick by placing their feet on the bottom of the tire and holding onto the top of the tire with their hands. The students then jump as if they had a Pogo stick.

If the inner tubes are available, have the bicycle shop save them as well. These tubes may be substituted for dynabands that are used for developing upper body strength. The tubes also are great for banding equipment such as bats together for easy storage.

Several activities and games require bicycle tires as the primary equipment. Not only are these games fun, they are also easy to set up. These games are great for transporting outside when the weather is nice.

UPPER BODY STRENGTH DEVELOPMENT ACTIVITIES

Bicycle tires may be used for some activities that can develop upper body strength. These activities include the following:

1. Take a push-up position with both hands in the tire. Walk around the tire using only the toes. Then reverse the direction of travel.

2. Take a push-up position with only one hand in the tire. Walk around the tire using only the toes. Then reverse the direction of travel.

3. Take a push-up position with both of the feet inside of the tire. Travel around the tire using only the hands. Then reverse the direction of travel.

4. Place both hands on the rim of the tire, take a push-up position, and travel around the tire using both the hands and the feet. Then reverse the direction of travel.

BICYCLE TIRE DODGE BALL

The students are placed in groups of three. Each group needs a bicycle tire and some sort of ball. This ball may be a panty hose ball, a Nerf ball, a boingo ball, a yarn ball, or other soft ball that will not sting if a student is struck with one. The dodger must stand inside the bicycle tire while the two throwers face each other from opposite sides of the tire. The distance between the throwers and the tire is approximately 12 feet. It may be less if a lightweight ball is used. The dodger is required to keep at least one foot inside of the tire. The two throwers try to hit the dodger no higher than the waist. If a thrower successfully strikes the dodger with a ball, the thrower takes the place of the dodger inside the tire and play resumes.

BICYCLE TIRE RACE

Each racing team should consist of two or three members so that they have just enough time to catch their breath before running again. This game is best for children who are in the third grade or older. This game requires five bicycle tires per team and one bean bag per player. The tires are placed in a line with approximately three feet between each tire. The teams stand in a line facing the five tires. The bean bags are all placed in the first tire. At the starting signal, the first player on the team runs to the first tire, picks up a bean bag, and weaves around the tires and back to the first tire. As the player runs around the last tire in the line, he or she drops the bean bag into the last tire. When the player returns to the first tire, he or she picks up a bean bag and hands it to the next player in the line. The first team to successfully transfer all of their bean bags to the last tire wins the game.

A variation of this game is to have the players transfer all of the bean bags back to the first tire again in the same manner that they were delivered to the last tire. The first team to transport all of their bean bags from the first tire to the last tire and back to the first tire again would be considered the winner

RESCUE THE TEACHER

This game requires a great number of old bicycle tires, but it is a hilariously fun game. The children are divided into four teams that each stand in one of the four corners of the room. The teacher stands in a tire that is placed in the center of the floor, which represents a small island in a large body of water. Each child holds a tire and many extra tires are placed behind the group for future use. At the sound of the starting signal, the first player tosses the tire on the floor ahead of him or her. The player steps into the tire with both feet, turns around, returns to the starting place, tags the next player, and then goes to the end of the line. The remaining players step through all of the tires that have been placed on the floor by the previous players, toss their tires down, and then repeat the action of the first player.

The first player to reach the teacher and successfully guide him through the tires and back to the team determines the winning team. If a player should step out of a tire and land in the water, that player must return to the starting point and begin again. A variation of this game is to have all teams on one end of the room and the teacher positioned at the opposite end of the room. This variation may work better for smaller gyms or rooms.

POPCORN BUCKETS

Visit the local theaters to see whether they would donate some of the buckets in which the largest size of popcorn is sold. Buckets in which fried chicken is sold would also be suitable for this activity. Students in groups of four or five use these buckets to cooperatively work together to build a fort. The forts should be located around the room in a circle. When the forts have been built, the students throw panty hose balls or tennis balls at the other forts to try to knock them over, while defending and repairing their own forts.

SECTION 2

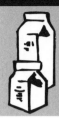

Equipment to Acquire by Collecting Proofs of Purchase

All of the offers presented in this section were current at the time of the writing of this book. Manufacturers, however, have the option of changing or deleting any programs that offer free equipment or cash to schools. The longer the program has been in existence, the better the odds are that it will continue to remain in existence with relatively few changes. Also, the longer a program has been around, the more problems have been worked out. All of these programs offer some wonderful and expensive equipment.

The best strategy to use when implementing programs such as these is to go slowly. Adding all of the programs in a single year would be overwhelming to the parents in the school. They would likely give up trying to save proofs of purchase because there would be so many items to save that they would begin to get confused. A good idea is to pick one or two programs that truly meet the needs of the school and implement those programs. When the parents have fully adopted those programs (it usually takes about a year or two), then another program may be incorporated.

Setting goals for a program when it is first established is also important to its success. Keeping the children, the parents, and the community aware of the progress made toward those goals is imperative to success. Often when a program is very near to reaching its goal, the community will rally and reach the goal. The key to this achievement is, of course, communication with the participants.

Along with the basic information about each program, some suggestions are given about methods of attaining extra labels or proofs of purchase. For any program, the more publicity that is done, the better the program will do. If the community is involved, the program will succeed. Once the school introduces the program, several public collection areas should be established. Collection boxes or canisters should be neatly made and attractive so that they call attention to themselves. They should be placed in areas where the general public visits or feels comfortable stopping to deposit labels. Some great places for collection canisters are public libraries, grocery stores, community recreation facilities, utility companies, and churches.

Once collection areas have been established, the newspapers should receive a press release that describes the program. The press release should indicate where the collection boxes are located in the community for residents that may not have any school-age children, but would be willing to donate the needed proofs of purchase to assist the school. The goals should be advertised so that people know why they are donating labels and will understand how they have helped the children. Most of the programs furnish press releases and parent letters that merely need to have specifics placed into the letter before sending them. The sponsoring corporation tries to make advertising as easy as possible for the coordinator of the program so that the program will be a success for both the school and the corporation.

CAMPBELL'S LABELS FOR EDUCATION

The Campbell's Labels for Education program was established in 1973 and runs very smoothly. Because this program has been around for so long, many people who have never participated in this program are aware that it exists. The Campbell's company often advertises this program in the Sunday Supplement section of the newspaper along with coupons for their products. Many of the packages from the participating products are marked with Labels for Education. This program is open to preschools, schools from grades K-12, licensed day care centers, public libraries, and United States military installations.

PRODUCTS INVOLVED IN THE PROGRAM

Campbell's products include a wide variety of brand names. These brand names include the following:

- Campbell's (beans, soups, ramen noodles, spaghetti sauce, tomato juice)
- Early California (olives)
- Franco American (gravy and pasta)
- Marie's (croutons, dips, dressings, glazes)

- Milwaukee's (pickles)
- Open Pit (barbecue sauce)
- Pace (picante sauce, salsa)
- Pepperidge Farms (bakery products, goldfish, cookies, crackers, soups, gravy)
- Prego (spaghetti sauce)
- Swana (ramen soups)
- Swanson (soups, broths, frozen food products)
- V8 (vegetable juice)
- Vlasic (pickles, olives, peppers, sauerkraut, cherries)

AVAILABLE MERCHANDISE

Under the category of sports, many items are available. Merchandise includes baseballs, batting tees, equipment bags, line markers, basketballs, footballs, pumps, soccer balls, cones, playground balls, treds balls, cageballs, horseshoes, tumbling mats, scooter boards, shuffle board sets, street hockey nets, street hockey gear, table tennis tables, table tennis gear, bowling pins, badminton sets, jump ropes, stop watches, balance boards, parachutes, Frisbees, tunnels, low balance beams, co-oper blankets, roller racers, tug-of-war ropes, and aerobics steps. This catalog probably has the greatest amount of available physical education equipment and supplies of all the programs. Other areas in the catalog may also have items of interest to physical educators, such as outdoor megaphones or audio equipment.

BONUS PROGRAMS

The Labels for Education program often presents bonus offers where a school may redeem particular labels for a greater value. Schools may turn as few as 500 labels into a value as great as 10,000 labels. When new products are introduced to the market, one method that the Campbell's company uses to promote the items is to make them bonus items for the Labels for Education program. The school coordinators then encourage the parents to try the new products and send the labels to the school. The Campbell's company hopes that those who try the new products will continue to purchase these new items.

The Labels for Education program also provides many methods of obtaining certificates that are redeemable for labels. For example, this program has offered bonus certificates for publicizing the school's participation in the program with the local newspapers. They have had contests for the most unique local promotional ideas, with the winning ideas receiving bonus certificates redeemable as labels. On occasion, stores that have machines that print coupons pending the purchase of designated merchandise will also print bonus certificates for the purchases of Campbell's products. These coupons are often unpublicized, but they are sometimes promoted through newsletters to the school's label coordinator.

Local distributors of Campbell's products also give grocery stores bonus certificates when they run a promotion for Campbell's products. The promotion may be a floor display or an advertisement in the store's sale flier. Some stores offer drawings to give away these certificates. The manager of other stores may give these certificates directly to a school. You should meet the local grocery store managers and find out how they distribute these certificates. You may be able to get them just by asking the manager.

MAXIMIZING COLLECTION

To maximize the collection of these particular brands, first be certain that the cafeteria manager is aware of the participating brands. Often the cafeteria may be using products made by Campbell's. Next, be aware of local restaurants that offer a soup and salad bar. They may use Campbell's soups. Often pubs or bars may put goldfish or pretzels out for patrons to enjoy. These may be made by Pepperidge Farms, which is also a participating brand. Older people may not have younger children for whom they are saving the labels. A collection bin at the local senior citizens' gathering place may prove to benefit collection efforts.

Recycling centers that process cans are also great sources for labels. Most will not be willing to supply the manpower to remove the labels, but will be willing to allow a representative from the school to remove the labels that are involved. If glass or cardboard are also processed there, the possibilities of finding labels is greatly increased. A little publicity will go a long way with these centers. If possible, have the local newspaper take pictures of someone cutting labels for the school. This publicity will make the recycling center look great as they support the schools and protect the environment. It also provides some free advertisement for the recycling center.

ENROLLMENT OR ADDITIONAL INFORMATION

To obtain additional information or to enroll in the program, call toll-free 1-800-424-5331. The mailing address is Campbell's Labels For Education, Post Office Box 4552, Monticello, Minnesota 55565.

POWER OF PURCHASING PROGRAM

The Power of Purchasing program was created in 1994. The materials supplied are very well organized and easy to use. The coordinator's packet includes examples of promotional letters to the press and to the parents. This program is available to churches, schools, and other tax-exempt community organizations.

PRODUCTS INVOLVED IN THE PROGRAM

The corporations that sponsor this program are Hershey's, Hefty, and Kodak. The requirement for redemption is the universal product code, also known as the UPC, from any product made by those three companies. This program is easy to promote because the UPC is the only requirement, and the products are common.

AVAILABLE MERCHANDISE

Under the sports category, a variety of items may be found. These include baseballs, baseball gloves, catcher's protective gear, equipment bags, footballs, basketballs, equipment carts, soccer balls, volleyballs, playground balls, hockey sticks, street hockey goals, bases, air pumps, cones, tether balls, Frisbees, horseshoes, bocce sets, low balance beams, badminton sets, table tennis tables, tumbling mats, jump ropes, and parachutes. Audio and video equipment is also available in another section of the catalog.

BONUS PROGRAMS

The Power of Purchasing program has offered enrollment bonuses for early enrollment. They have periodically offered double points for particular items or early submission. These items may be submitted several times during the promotion.

MAXIMIZING COLLECTION

Often companies such as insurance companies or real estate companies are required to take pictures of properties or damages. Most companies would be willing to save empty film packages to assist the schools in obtaining needed equipment.

ENROLLMENT OR ADDITIONAL INFORMATION

To obtain additional information or to enroll in this program, the telephone number is 1-800-362-4648. The mailing address is Power of Purchasing Program, 9060 Zachary Lane North, Suite 111, Maple Grove, Minnesota 55311.

BOXTOPS FOR EDUCATION

The Boxtops for Education program ran as a pilot program in a handful of states starting in 1993. The program, which has changed names since it began as a pilot program, was introduced on a national basis in 1996. With the introduction of the program on a national basis, the packaging of the participating products has also changed to help heighten the awareness of the promotion. As a result, most people who use the products are aware that the proofs of purchase are valuable to schools. The excellent coordinator's package includes promotional letters to the parents in both English and Spanish, sample press releases, and classroom collection bags. The Boxtops for Education program has a narrower field of eligibility than some of the other programs. It is open to all accredited K-6 public, private, parochial, and military schools in the United States.

PRODUCTS INVOLVED IN THE PROGRAM

All General Mills cereals are eligible for redemption. The necessary proof of purchase is the boxtop that has the Boxtops for Education logo printed on it. The Betty Crocker points also printed on the boxtop with the logo are not necessary for redemption of the boxtop. Therefore, if you know someone collecting points, they can keep the points and you can still use the boxtop for this program. The participating cereals include Cheerios (any flavor), Cinnamon Toast

Crunch, Cocoa Puffs, Golden Grahams, Lucky Charms, Kix, Boo Berry, Count Chocula, S'mores, Trix, Reese's Peanut Butter Puffs, Triples, Kaboom, Oatmeal Crisp (any flavor), Raisin Nut Bran, Basic 4, Honey Nut Clusters, Fiber One, Nature Valley Low Fat Fruit Granola, Country Corn Flakes, Total, Wheaties, and Betty Crocker Dutch Apple or Cinnamon Streusel.

AVAILABLE MERCHANDISE

Each boxtop has a redemption value of 15 cents. This money may be spent any way that the school finds necessary. There are no restrictions for the spending of the money generated by this program.

BONUS PROGRAMS

A bonus of 50 dollars is given for every 750 boxtops that are redeemed. Although boxtops may be redeemed prior to the deadline of the program, the bonus is not sent until the deadline has passed.

MAXIMIZING COLLECTION

Many home day care providers use cereal as a staple food for the children. Some feed the children cereal for breakfast or for snacks nearly every day. They are usually cooperative people because they must have a patient nature to be successful day care providers. Most will be willing to save boxtops for a school if they are not eligible themselves because they do not have elementary school children of their own. You can locate many of these home day care providers through advertisements for child care in the newspapers.

The local WIC department may also be willing to let a school put a collection box and promotional materials there. Many of the participating cereals are on the approved cereal list for WIC participants. Placing a collection box at the facility where participants pick up their vouchers will aid in the collection of the boxtops.

ENROLLMENT OR ADDITIONAL INFORMATION

To acquire additional information or to enroll in this program, call toll-free 1-888-799-2444. You can also obtain information through the Internet at **http://www.boxtops4education.com.**

LITTLE DEBBIE POINTS TO EDUCATION PROGRAM

This program was piloted for seven years before going to a national level in 1996. It comes with a nice color catalog and promotional materials, including posters to show the progress of the collection. Schools, grades K-12, located in the continental United States are eligible to participate.

PRODUCTS INVOLVED IN THE PROGRAM

Labels from any Little Debbie or Sunbelt brand multipacks and cereals may be used in this program.

AVAILABLE MERCHANDISE

The equipment offered under the athletic section includes volleyballs, footballs, baseballs, soccer balls, playground balls, basketballs, portable basketball goals, soccer goals, baseball gloves, shin guards, tennis rackets, batting tees, hockey sticks, and baseball bats.

BONUS PROGRAMS

No bonus programs have been available in the past.

MAXIMIZING COLLECTION

Child care centers are likely to use these products. Because they are not eligible to participate in the program, they may be willing to save labels for a school that is eligible.

ENROLLMENT OR ADDITIONAL INFORMATION

You can get information about enrollment in the program by calling 1-800-619-3215. The mailing address is Points to Education Redemption Center, 3466 Holcomb Bridge Road, Suite 179, Norcross, Georgia 30092.

KIDS IN GEAR PROGRAM BY FUJI

This program started in 1994 in conjunction with Fuji's sponsorship of the World Cup. It was designed to assist children playing soccer to obtain team uniforms. Although the program was somewhat dormant in 1995, the program reappeared in 1996 with swimming and track and field added to the program. The unique element of this program is that it offers items, such as team jerseys and McDonald's gift certificates, that may not be found in other redemption catalogs. It comes with a nice handbook and color catalog. Also included are promotional letters to send to parents and to the newspapers. This program is directed toward soccer clubs, swim teams, and track and field teams. It is open to organizations and school teams located in the continental United States that are participating in a recognized or structured soccer, swimming, or track and field program.

PRODUCTS INVOLVED IN THE PROGRAM

All products made by Fuji are eligible for the program. These products are film, quicksnap cameras, floppy disks, audiocassettes, and videocassettes. Cut out the little squares on the back of the film packages that say 10 or 30 Fuji Kids in Gear points. Fuji requires the upc from floppy disks and audio or video tapes.

AVAILABLE MERCHANDISE

An unusual collection of merchandise is available through this catalog. These items include training videos, McDonald's gift certificates, cones, watches, gear bags, shin guards, soccer balls, pumps, shoe bags, denim jackets, hats, T-shirts, beach towels, swim caps, warm-up suits, cameras, polo shirts, sweatshirts, soccer jerseys, goalie shirts, and soccer shorts.

BONUS PROGRAMS

Bonus programs have not been available.

MAXIMIZING COLLECTION

As with Kodak film, any real estate companies or insurance companies that use film in the operation of their businesses would be great sources for additional proofs of purchase.

ENROLLMENT OR ADDITIONAL INFORMATION

You can contact this organization by calling 1-800-543-1032. The mailing address is Kids in Gear, Post Office Box 1411, Ridgely, Maryland 21681.

OTHER PROGRAMS THAT MAY BE AVAILABLE

Many other companies have sponsored similar redemption programs on a smaller scale. Castrol oil has offered free footballs with the purchase of a case of oil. Energizer has offered several promotions where battery UPCs were redeemable for baseballs, baseball jerseys, soccer balls, or other sports items. Lipton tea had a redemption offer for fox tails. Cereal boxes often have redemption programs to obtain Frisbees, Koosh balls, target games, or other small items such as water bottles. Green Giant offered a program where the UPCs from their vegetables could be redeemed for Little Sprout jump ropes. Crest and Scope gave soccer balls for their proofs of purchase. Pepsi had miniature balls that came three in a set with a carrying bag that could be purchased with Pepsi points.

The easiest way to find out about these redemption programs is to watch for specially marked packages. Slow down as you wander through the grocery aisles and look for the word *Free* written on packages. Some stores keep a special bulletin board for forms for redemption. Most K-mart stores, for example, have such a board. Check these boards periodically for new offers that may be interesting. These offers occur sporadically. When they are spotted, they are usually worth investigating. Sometimes, special offers may require a handling fee. Usually this fee is much smaller than the cost of the item. If you were to purchase the item through an equipment company, it would probably carry a postage and handling fee that would be similar to the one required in a redemption program.

Beware! These redemption programs are exciting and can become addicting! Once the free items begin to pour in, the person ordering them may want to find more and more programs. Fortunately, they are usually available.

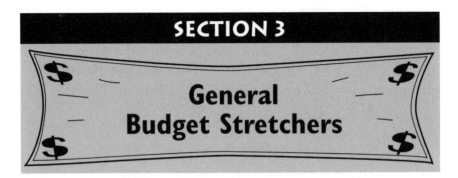

SECTION 3

General
Budget Stretchers

There are many methods of stretching a physical education budget. Not all of them will work for every program, but utilizing even one budget stretching idea will help economize and supply additional equipment.

Manufacturer's display booths, which are often located at state or national physical education conventions, usually have 10 percent discount certificates available for the taking. They may be located with the catalogs or set out separately. Do not hesitate to ask one of the representatives for them if they are not clearly visible. Often at the end of one of these conventions, the company will sell the items that were on display at a very reasonable price. They would prefer to sell these items so that they do not have to pack them and ship them home. If an item does not appear to be selling for the price marked on it, make an offer for it. The representative may take it to keep from taking it back home. If a purchase order is required and making purchases on a spur of the moment basis at a convention is not a possibility, do not just order from a catalog. Speak to a representative and ask what discount can be given. Often, a dealer will give a 10 percent discount just for the asking. No catalog form will be able to do this.

If funds for equipment are not available, swapping equipment with another physical education teacher is a possibility. If one school has tumbling mats and another school has portable volleyball standards, they may swap them for a few weeks. This system enhances the programs for both of the schools. Get to know other local teachers and find out what is available for trading.

Recreation departments may be a source of assistance when equipment is needed. If a school needs to borrow tumbling mats, the recreation program may be willing to lend some in exchange for advertisement for their gymnastics program. At the conclusion of the tumbling unit, a small flier that tells about the available gymnastics programs at the recreation center may be given to the children. Those who enjoyed the tumbling unit may want to enroll in the recreation department's program to continue learning more difficult tumbling. This free advertising benefits the recreation program as well as benefiting the physical education program by allowing more opportunities for learning.

Recreation departments may also be willing to swap equipment for space. If they need a facility to teach tumbling or to have volleyball competitions, they may leave the necessary equipment at the school. The school would be allowed to use the equipment for physical education classes in exchange for allowing the recreation department to use the space on Saturday mornings. This situation enhances both programs.

CHAPTER 6

FUNDRAISING

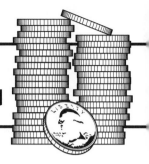

No matter how much equipment is donated, created, or adapted, there will always be items such as expensive gymnastic equipment, uniforms, or track and field landing mats that are extremely expensive and may be beyond the budget of a physical education program. If a school is to acquire such expensive equipment, fundraising has to be done. Fundraising is often a painful and dreaded process for physical educators who are already involved with teaching and coaching responsibilities. However, fundraising does not have to be time-consuming and painful. There are many methods of earning money that will consume very little time from the administrator of the fundraising program.

This chapter is divided into two sections. The first section deals with fundraising activities that are called "painless" fundraisers. These activities require very little time and organization from the sponsor of the activity. They do not require solicitation by the students, and they do not require the parents to buy any items that are outrageously priced. They also require very little paperwork for the sponsor. Some are ongoing activities that last throughout the school year and possibly through the summer. These activities bring in funds slowly, but they are steady, dependable income producers. The parents will gladly support these painless fundraisers because very little work and no solicitation is required from them. With children involved in selling items through their churches, scout groups, parent-teacher organizations, athletic teams, and a variety of other activities in which their children participate, the parents will appreciate this painless approach.

The second section deals with fundraisers that are a little more painful. These fundraisers require more organizational time from the sponsor of the activity and may require some solicitation on the part of the participants. These activities go beyond the basic bake sale into something somewhat more unique. Their unusual nature may help the parents be more willing to allow the students to participate because they will not be "burned out" on these activities.

Before you begin any fundraising program, make sure that you discuss your plan with a school administrator. He or she should ensure that your plan is consistent with the school's policy and in some cases he or she may have a lawyer review the plan for any inconsistencies with policy. Many states have detailed requirements to keep fundraising efforts honest, and it's best to make sure your program is both legal and consistent with school policy *before* you start.

SECTION 1

Painless Fundraisers

In all physical education programs, one thing is certain, funds will be needed. Equipment will wear out, get lost, or break during the year. Uniforms will wear out or disappear and need to be replaced. Another thing is also certain, parents and coaches tire of traditional fundraising tactics that require a lot of time, effort, and solicitation. The fundraising ideas presented in this section of the chapter will be invigorating to parents and coaches who have been involved in other forms of fundraising. In comparison, these tactics are less time-consuming and refreshingly creative.

RECYCLING

Some companies will make this recycling project extremely easy. The sponsor simply calls the recycling company to have bins for newspaper and aluminum cans placed on the campus. (Some communities may recycle other materials such as plastic and steel as well.) When the bin is full, the sponsor calls the company to pick it up, and the company writes a check to the school for the amount of weight that was in the bin. This ongoing project can run through the summer. It doesn't generate funds quickly, but it does provide a steady source of income.

In some areas, this project may not be as simple as using the telephone. Some areas require the materials that are being recycled to be delivered by the sponsor of the program. If the sponsor does not have a vehicle that will transport the materials, a parent volunteer who has a truck, van, or trailer will need to be solicited to help with the project. With either method, the children learn an outstanding lesson about protecting their environment while generating income for the school.

RESTAURANT NIGHTS

Many restaurants, such as McDonald's and Pizza Inn, sponsor group nights. The school gives out certificates that state the night and the time that the participants may go to the restaurant for credit for the school. The restaurant collects the certificates as the participants order. The total of the order is written on the certificate. At the end of the specified time period, the certificates are gathered and totaled. A percentage of the money collected is given to the school or group.

Parents who do the cooking will enjoy having this fundraiser as an excuse to eat out. They do not have to pay any additional fees for eating, and the school benefits. Many restaurants will be willing to make this an ongoing event. For example, the first Monday of every month could be your school's night. It will be beneficial to make this night one that is just after pay day for most people.

GROCERY VOUCHERS

Some national chain grocery stores, such as Food Lion and Kroger, sponsor programs for generating funds for nonprofit organizations. One program involves the school selecting three consecutive days to be their voucher days. Each parent is given four vouchers to use or to give to friends and neighbors. If a parent shops on one of those three days, the parent gives the voucher to the cashier. The cashier writes the amount spent on the voucher and turns it in to the office with the cash drawer at the end of the shift. All vouchers are totaled at the end of the three days and the school is given 5 percent of the total amount that was spent. The parents enjoy this fundraiser because they already buy groceries. Some may have to change the day that they normally shop, but this is a minor inconvenience for most. They would much rather shop on a different day than spend countless hours at car washes or bake sales.

Some franchised grocery stores already have these programs available for the asking. Small or local grocery stores may be willing to participate in a program of this nature if the owner were presented with a proposal outlining the details. They benefit by having the opportunity to have some new customers try their store and by getting some free advertising. Have the owner or manager of the store come to the school to get his or her picture in the paper presenting a check to the school. This kind of event makes some wonderful public relations for the store involved in the program.

CONSIGNMENT CLOTHING

At the end of the year, instead of giving the clothing that has been left in the lost and found to a charity or throwing it out, take it to a consignment store. The clothes will need to be washed before being presented to the store. You can do this at the school with school machines and soap during the post-planning days. This activity will not generate great amounts of money, but it may generate enough to buy some new balls or racquets.

VENDING MACHINES

If there are no vending machines in the faculty lounge, you could have some installed. Most soda or snack companies will keep them supplied and send a check for a percentage of the profits. Machines may also be placed near the gym for times when the gym is used after regular school hours. Many gyms are used by community groups and do not provide concessions. These machines could be unplugged during school hours if the school is not allowed to sell these items to students during school hours.

NO-WORK CAR WASH

You can do this fundraiser in a few different ways. A local full-serve car wash may issue certificates so that when a customer gets a car wash and redeems the certificate, the school gets 50 cents. At the end of each month, the car wash sends a check to the school. The students should take home one of these certificates every month.

You could also do this fundraiser as a frequent car wash club. The parents would be issued a card that would be punched every time they have their cars washed. When the card has been punched 10 times, the school would receive credit for five dollars. The car wash would tally the credits and write a check to the school every three months.

A third method of the no-work car wash is to have credit vouchers at the car wash. Each time someone from the school visits the car wash, that customer picks up a voucher. The vouchers are turned in to the school, and the school redeems them every three months at the car wash. Parents who use a full-service car wash may be willing to try the particular car wash that supports the school. This fundraiser could introduce new customers to the business while earning money for the school.

TEST DRIVE

Some car dealerships are willing to pay for test drivers. Parents who take a certificate with the school's name on it to the dealership on a certain day or weekend can earn credit for the school. The school and the dealership set up a point system. Every test driver earns one point. The points may be redeemed for money or for equipment, depending upon the dealership involved. In addition, the dealership will probably be willing to give a bonus of $50 or $100 for anyone who buys a vehicle as a result of this promotion. All parents and faculty members are eligible to test drive the cars. Although this fundraiser does take a little of their time, many people will be willing to participate because they don't have to put out any cash toward this fundraiser. Many are willing to give some time to help, but most get tired of donating money or buying items that they truly do not need or could buy elsewhere for half the price.

SECTION 2

Fundraisers That Are a Little Painful

These fundraisers involve a little more time, cost an admission fee, or require some solicitation. Be sure to utilize parent volunteers for these fundraisers. They can be ticket takers, coupon cutters, or other helpful workers.

SHOW IN THE GYM

The show could be a local clown, magician, or entertainer. This show could also be a game of the faculty versus the students or the parents of the students. The admission price should be low so that attendance will be great. If the admission fee is 50 cents, most of the students probably will be able to attend. If possible, hold the show during school hours. With a low admission fee, nearly every student in the school would be able to attend. Try to get the local celebrity to donate his or her time in exchange for free advertising. For example, the clown may want to send home a business card with the students that says the clown is available for birthday parties. The extra business that the clown could get would more than "pay" for the show performed at the school.

VALENTINE SERENADE

This fundraiser involves contacting all of the spouses or "significant others" of the teachers. For a fee of three or five dollars, a group of children will appear at the teacher's door and sing "You Are My Sunshine," replacing "sunshine" with "Valentine."

The students knock on the teacher's door while the teacher is in the middle of a class and announce that they are to present a singing valentine from whomever sent the valentine. They then proceed to sing the song. This is a great method of generating funds because there is no need to buy anything to hold this event. All of the money that is earned is clear profit. This fundraiser involves a little practice with the children who are going to serenade and some time to contact the ones who are to purchase the valentines. To keep the singing valentine a surprise, the sponsor may offer to bill the spouse after the valentine has been delivered.

DOG WASH

Instead of holding a car wash, hold a dog wash. After about two hours of washing the dogs, a dog show may be held. Charge a fee for washing the dogs, and hold the dog show as a free bonus for attending. The dog show may be serious, or it may have a fun tone to it by awarding ribbons for the scruffiest dog, the dog that looks most like its owner, the biggest dog, the smallest dog, or the ugliest dog. You can make the ribbons by hanging strips of paper on a large dog treat or bone.

TEACHER OF THE YEAR: STUDENTS' CHOICE

Jars with pictures of every teacher and administrator attached to them are placed in the library or other common area of the school. For a week, children drop spare change into them. The teacher or administrator who has the most money in his or her jar at the end of the week is selected as the Teacher of the Year at the next pep assembly or parent-teacher meeting. The last day to place money in the jars should also be the day of the event. If the event is to be held at the parent-teacher meeting, the jars could be available before the meeting so that the parents also can place money into the jars. This activity could also be done at half time of a ball game. The jars could be available throughout the first quarter of the game, and the teacher could be announced at the halftime period.

BIRTHDAY CUPCAKES

This fundraiser may be a lot of work, but it is often very popular. The sponsor sends a note home to all parents offering to deliver a dozen cupcakes to their children on their birthdays. For an additional two dollars, a group of students could sing "Happy Birthday" to the child when the cupcakes are delivered. The cost of the cupcakes depends upon the price of the cupcakes from a local bakery or grocery with a bakery. They may give a discount to the school as a nonprofit organization or because of the high number of cupcakes that will be needed through the year. The note should be sent at the beginning of the year and all money collected then. The sponsor would then have the money in an account to buy the cupcakes and would be able to make a calendar showing all of the needed cupcakes and serenades. The bakery then could have ample notice for the necessary cupcakes.

In order that new students who enroll after school has started are not eliminated from this activity, a special flier describing the activity should be drafted. One of the fliers, with the information of how to submit the money for this event included on the flier, should be given to the parents along with any other vital information given at the time of enrollment. A notice could also be placed in the student handbook that all students receive at the beginning of the year or upon enrollment. Many parents will be grateful to not have to bake the cupcakes, and many students are reaching an age where they would be embarrassed if a parent showed up at school to deliver cupcakes. The cupcakes could be delivered during lunch so that class instruction is not interrupted.

SCHOOL DANCE

A dance is a relatively easy fundraiser to hold. If a teacher or parent has the equipment and is willing to play music, the expenses will be minimal. Concessions may be sold at the dance to earn an additional profit. Polaroid pictures at the dance are also popular. By charging a rate of two dollars per picture, you can make nearly 100 percent profit. If charging an admission fee is a problem, the students could be admitted for aluminum cans, cereal boxtops, Campbell's labels, newspapers, or other items that are currently being used to trade for equipment or cash. This dance could be the kick-off for a collection program. Be sure to give the parents enough notice so that they may buy and consume the item that is necessary for admission to the dance.

GRANTS

Do not overlook possible grants. Many school systems offer mini-grants for innovative projects. Come up with a new teaching technique or tie a physical education lesson in with a classroom teacher's objectives. Then apply for the grant to purchase the equipment necessary to carry out the project. Do not be discouraged if a grant proposal is rejected. Look for another source of grant money and resubmit the proposal.

Look through professional journals to find grants that are currently available. The Internet may also be a source of grant information. Professional associations may also be aware of grants that are available in the physical education field. There may be an employee of the local Board of Education that oversees grant writing projects. This person may be aware of available money. If you can't find any formal grants, you can draw up a proposal and give it to one of the local service clubs. The Kiwanis, Knights of Columbus, Women's Club or other local organization may have money that may be allotted for educational projects. Sometimes getting the money merely requires that you ask and apply for it.

POWDERPUFF FOOTBALL

A very popular event where schools have football teams and cheerleading squads is called powderpuff football. The football players are all female, and the cheerleaders are all male. This role reversal will prove to be an entertaining event. The teams need to organize themselves and practice a little before the game. The cheerleaders should meet with the cheerleading sponsor or one of the cheerleaders to prepare some cheers for the game. If possible, the faculty could do a special halftime show. One of the teachers could be crowned as the "Powderpuff Fossil." This title could be voted upon by the students of the school. To make money, sell tickets for this event. A special price may be given to those who pay in advance, and tickets at the door could be a little more expensive. For additional revenue, parent volunteers could sell concessions at the game.

BIBLIOGRAPHY

Lyons, Russell and Kermit R. Davis. *"Homemade" Equipment That Can Be Used in Teaching Physical Education Classes.* Jackson, Mississippi; State Department of Education.

Stier, William F. 1994. *Fundraising for Sport and Recreation.* Champaign, Illinois: Human Kinetics.

Stillwell, Jim L. 1987. *Making and Using Creative Play Equipment.* Champaign, Illinois: Human Kinetics.

INDEX
OF GAMES

ABOUT THE AUTHOR

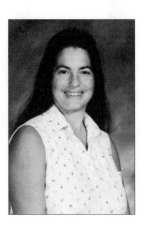

Bev Davison is a veteran physical educator, having taught for ten years at the elementary and secondary levels. During those years she mastered the skill of creating a quality physical education program on a shoestring budget. She has shared her knowledge on this subject with fellow physical educators far and wide—from the Georgia Association for Health, Physical Education, Recreation and Dance (GAHPERD) state convention to a naval base in Cuba.

One of Davison's most significant career accomplishments was being named the 1995-96 Teacher of the Year by fellow teachers at her school for implementing the ideas in this book. Davison's contributions to her school's physical education program also led to a 1996 School of Excellence in Physical Education Honorable Mention Award from GAHPERD.

Davison is a member of the American Alliance for Health, Physical Education, Recreation and Dance and GAHPERD. She earned her master's degree in physical education from Eastern Kentucky University. In her free time she enjoys biking, fishing, and water sports. She and her husband, Ray, live in St. Mary's, Georgia, with their three children.

More Games Books from Human Kinetics

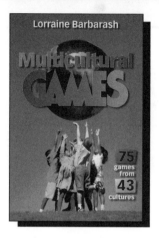

Lorraine Barbarash

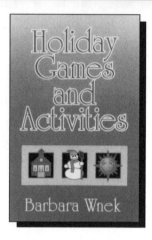

Barbara Wnek

An excellent source for ideas on building an interdisciplinary and multicultural curriculum at the elementary and middle school level. Features 75 games from 43 countries or cultures on 6 continents.

1997 • Paper • 152 pp
Item BBAR0565 • ISBN 0-88011-565-3
$14.95 ($21.95 Canadian)

Promote holiday spirit in your classes while providing quality physical education for kids in kindergarten through grade 6. Loaded with physical fitness activities, skills, games, rhythm and dance activities, and illustrated bulletin board ideas for each holiday or season.

1992 • Paper • 184 pp
Item BWNE0355 • ISBN 0-87322-355-1
$14.95 ($21.95 Canadian)

Human Kinetics offers a wide variety of physical education games books and teaching resources! For a FREE copy of our current physical education catalog, call us or visit our Web site TODAY!

Prices subject to change.

HUMAN KINETICS
The Information Leader in Physical Activity
http: // www.humankinetics.com /

For more information or to place your order, U.S. customers
call toll-free 1-800-747-4457.
Customers outside the U.S. use the appropriate telephone number/address shown in the front of this book.